Neuropathology

Editor

TARIK TIHAN

SURGICAL PATHOLOGY CLINICS

www.surgpath.theclinics.com

Consulting Editor
JOHN R. GOLDBLUM

March 2015 • Volume 8 • Number 1

ELSEVIER

1600 John F. Kennedy Boulevard • Suite 1800 • Philadelphia, Pennsylvania, 19103-2899

http://www.theclinics.com

SURGICAL PATHOLOGY CLINICS Volume 8, Number 1
March 2015 ISSN 1875-9181, ISBN-13: 978-0-323-39208-2

Editor: Joanne Husovski
Developmental Editor: Donald Mumford

Surgical Pathology Clinics (ISSN 1875-9181) is published quarterly by Elsevier Inc., 360 Park Avenue South, New York, NY 10010. Months of issue are March, June, September, and December. Business and Editorial Office: Elsevier Inc., 1600 John F. Kennedy Blvd., Ste. 1800, Philadelphia, PA 19103-2899. Accounting and Circulation Offices: Elsevier Inc., 3251 Riverport Lane, Maryland Heights, MO 63043. Periodicals postage paid at New York, NY and at additional mailing offices. Subscription prices are $200.00 per year (US individuals), $233.00 per year (US institutions), $100.00 per year (US students/residents), $250.00 per year (Canadian individuals), $266.00 per year (Canadian Institutions), $250.00 per year (foreign individuals), $266.00 per year (foreign institutions), and $120.00 per year (international & Canadian students/residents). Foreign air speed delivery is included in all *Clinics'* subscription prices. All prices are subject to change without notice. **POSTMASTER:** Send address changes to *Surgical Pathology Clinics*, Elsevier, 3251 Riverport Lane, Maryland Heights, MO 63043. Customer Service: 1-800-654-2452 (US). From outside the United States, call 1-314-447-8871. Fax: 1-314-447-8029. E-mail: JournalsCustomerServiceusa@elsevier.com (for print support) and JournalsOnlineSupport-usa@elsevier.com (for online support).

Reprints. For copies of 100 or more, of articles in this publication, please contact the Commercial Reprints Department, Elsevier Inc., 360 Park Avenue South, New York, NY 10010-1710. Tel. 212-633-3874; Fax: 212-633-3820; E-mail: reprints@elsevier.com.

Contributors

CONSULTING EDITOR

JOHN R. GOLDBLUM, MD
Chairman, Professor of Pathology, Department
of Anatomic Pathology, Cleveland Clinics
Lerner College of Medicine, Cleveland Clinic,
Cleveland, Ohio

EDITOR

TARIK TIHAN, MD, PhD
Professor of Pathology, Neuropathology
Division, Department of Pathology,
UCSF Medical Center, UCSF School of
Medicine, University of California, San
Francisco, San Francisco, California

AUTHORS

GREGORY FULLER, MD, PhD
Neuropathology Division, Department of
Pathology, UCSF School of Medicine,
San Francisco, California; University of
Texas MD Anderson Cancer Center,
Houston, Texas

CHRISTINE M. GLASTONBURY, MBBS
Department of Radiology and Biomedical
Imaging, UCSF School of Medicine, San
Francisco, California

S. HUMAYUN GULTEKIN, MD
Associate Professor, Department of Pathology,
Oregon Health and Science University,
Portland, Oregon

HAN S. LEE, MD, PhD
Assistant Professor of Pathology,
Neuropathology Division, Department of
Anatomic Pathology, University of California,
San Francisco, San Francisco, California

MELIKE PEKMEZCI, MD
Clinical Fellow, Division of Neuropathology,
Department of Pathology, University of
California, San Francisco, San Francisco,
California

ARIE PERRY, MD
Director of Neuropathology, Division of
Neuropathology; Professor of Pathology,
Department of Pathology; Professor of
Neurosurgery, Department of
Neurological Surgery, University of
California, San Francisco, San Francisco,
California

JOANNA PHILLIPS, MD, PhD
Neuropathology Division, Department of
Pathology, UCSF School of Medicine,
UCSF Medical Center, San Francisco,
California

GERALD F. REIS, MD, PhD
Neuropathology Division, Department of
Pathology, UCSF School of Medicine, San
Francisco, California

TARIK TIHAN, MD, PhD
Professor of Pathology, Neuropathology
Division, Department of Pathology, UCSF
School of Medicine, UCSF Medical Center,
University of California, San Francisco,
San Francisco, California

Contents

Imaging has established itself as an irreplaceable component of neuro-oncology,
and provided much insight in all aspects of central nervous system (CNS) tumors.
Today, similar to some other medical specialties, such as bone and joint disorders,
it is an integral part of the diagnosis of CNS tumors. This brief review highlights the
critical elements of neuroimaging, especially of MRI, in the study and diagnosis of
brain tumors, and considers some of the common entities for the diagnosis, of which
a good understanding of imaging characteristics is extremely helpful.

Intraoperative pathologic consultation continues to be an essential tool during
neurosurgical procedures, helping to ensure adequacy of material for achieving a
pathologic diagnosis and to guide surgeons. For pathologists, successful consultation with central nervous system lesions involves not only a basic familiarity with the
pathologic features of such lesions but also an understanding of their clinical and
radiologic context. This review discusses a basic approach to intraoperative diagnosis for practicing pathologists, including preparation for, performance of, and
interpretation of an intraoperative neuropathologic evaluation. The cytologic and
frozen section features of select examples of common pathologic entities are
described.

Recent advances in molecular diagnostics have led to better understanding of glioma tumorigenesis and biology. Numerous glioma biomarkers with diagnostic,
prognostic, and predictive value have been identified. Although some of these
markers are already part of the routine clinical management of glioma patients,
data regarding others are limited and difficult to apply routinely. In addition, multiple
methods for molecular subclassification have been proposed either together with or
as an alternative to the current morphologic classification and grading scheme. This
article reviews the literature regarding glioma biomarkers and offers a few practical
suggestions.

The pilocytic astrocytoma is predominantly a tumor of childhood and the most common type of circumscribed astrocytoma. The indolent nature of this tumor allows for
prolonged survival for most patients, rendering the disease a rather "chronic" one,

SURGICAL PATHOLOGY CLINICS

Preface

Practical Issues in Diagnostic Neuropathology: It Is Not Even the End of the Beginning!

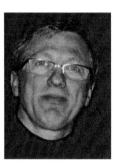

Tarik Tihan, MD, PhD
Editor

Classification schemes are often dynamic, living paradigms that periodically undergo expansion or shrinkage, fragmentation or coherence, and yet, inescapably become more comprehensive and multidimensional. What started as mere interpretations of the light microscopic images in the last century are now facing significant modifications through the use of a spectrum of advanced analytical tools. Classification of the diseases of the central nervous system (CNS), and in particular, tumors and paraneoplastic diseases, is no exception. The last two decades have seen tremendous progress in advanced technology, such as MRI and molecular biology, and it is no longer possible to ignore the wealth of information provided by these technologies in the understanding, diagnosis, and treatment of CNS diseases.

Until a decade ago, it was mostly sufficient to provide the type and the grade of a CNS neoplasm based on the routine H&E stains alone, and this bit of information was helpful in an overwhelming majority of tumors. In fact, the neuro-oncologists did not have specific treatment for most of the tumor types or variants in the WHO classification scheme. Some entities, variants, or families of tumors were being managed in the same fashion, so a lengthy debate about whether a neoplasm should be considered oligoastrocytoma or astrocytoma was only relevant at the microscope, but not at the bedside. Our occasionally subjective

interpretations and discrepancies in neuropathology were of little consequence, and the pathologic interpretation was useful as long as it gave the treating physician a general idea on the nature of the disease.

Well, that era is over! It has been brought to an end by the expanding number of advanced treatment options, diagnostic methodologies, and the attempts to "personalize" patient management. It is time to recognize the complexities of biology that give us a spectrum of genotypic and phenotypic attributes of the same pathologic process and to give equal importance to both. It is still critical to recognize the phenotypic attributes of a disease as reflected under the microscope. Yet, mere phenotypic characterization is increasingly becoming incomplete as we understand the other side of the coin. It is time for the pathologists to add a few more weapons to their diagnostic arsenal other than the faithful light microscope.

The articles in this issue of *Surgical Pathology Clinics* are a testament to the fact that characterization of tumors above and beyond the information provided on routine histological stains is no longer a feat of "fancy" academic centers alone. Today, the practicing pathologists have to incorporate the information that was mostly limited to reports from advanced academic centers only a decade ago. It is with this realization that the authors in this issue have provided their expertise

Surgical Pathology 8 (2015) ix–x
http://dx.doi.org/10.1016/j.path.2014.12.001

surgpath.theclinics.com

and experience to practicing pathologists at all levels.

The first article by Glastonbury et al is a gentle warning to practicing pathologists that neuropathologic interpretation can be significantly aided by a good understanding of neuroradiology, which can be achieved through collaboration with a neuroradiologist. The importance of intraoperative consultation and how it can be practiced with the utmost benefit to the patients are highlighted in the article by Lee. The articles by Pekmezci et al and by Reis et al underscore the need to include a set of critical molecular markers in the diagnosis of both diffuse and solid glial neoplasms. The markers detailed in these articles are no longer "luxury items" and will need to be available for the upcoming standard of care in surgical neuropathology. Substantive changes in the understanding of diffuse glial neoplasm are imminent, and these will provide a significant modification of the existing WHO 2007 scheme. Phillips and colleagues briefly summarize the impressive amount of progress on embryonal tumors that took place in the last few years. It is important to recognize the markers that will be asked of the practicing pathologists when reporting CNS embryonal tumors. Finally, Dr Gultekin, a world expert in the diagnosis and evaluation of paraneoplastic diseases in the CNS, provides a comprehensive and enlightening review of these enigmatic entities. His tables and figures are very helpful in understanding the new developments, and the article provides a beautiful template for aiding the workup of these challenging entities.

I am deeply indebted to all the authors for the time and the effort they have put into this issue. I also wish to acknowledge the hundreds of excellent scientists who have reported their results in numerous publications, recent or remote. Without their collective effort of adding one building block of information at a time, we would have little, if any, understanding of the mechanisms of CNS diseases, their pathogenesis, treatment, or prognosis. I feel proud to be able to work with all the authors to bring a synopsis of these advances to our readers. This feeling was best formulated a few centuries ago by Sir Isaac Newton: *"If I have seen further, it is by standing on the shoulders of giants."* We can look further ahead together to see what is beyond the next hill.

Tarik Tihan, MD, PhD
Neuropathology Division
Department of Pathology
UCSF School of Medicine
UCSF Medical Center
Room M551
505 Parnassus Avenue
San Francisco
CA 94143-0102, USA

E-mail address:
Tarik.Tihan@ucsf.edu

Practical Neuroimaging of Central Nervous System Tumors for Surgical Pathologists

Christine M. Glastonbury, MBBS[a], Tarik Tihan, MD, PhD[b],*

KEYWORDS

• CNS tumors • Neuroimaging • Neuro-oncology • CNS metastases

ABSTRACT

Imaging has established itself as an irreplaceable component of neuro-oncology, and provided much insight in all aspects of central nervous system (CNS) tumors. Today, similar to some other medical specialties, such as bone and joint disorders, it is an integral part of the diagnosis of CNS tumors. This brief review highlights the critical elements of neuroimaging, especially of MRI, in the study and diagnosis of brain tumors, and considers some of the common entities for the diagnosis, of which a good understanding of imaging characteristics is extremely helpful.

OVERVIEW: YOU CAN'T HAVE ONE WITHOUT THE OTHER!

Over the past 4 decades, the medical world has witnessed impressive progress in disease diagnosis and treatment with the aid of basic sciences, such as physics and chemistry. Some of the greatest advances have been recorded in the field of imaging, with the discovery and rapid development of computerized tomography (CT) and MRI of the human body. The more detailed imaging obtained through multiple modalities has improved our understanding of disease, allowed more precise diagnoses, treatment monitoring, and a greater degree of accuracy in determining prognosis.

Specifically, neuroimaging has provided critical information for the diagnosis and treatment of central nervous system (CNS) diseases. Today, it is virtually impossible to imagine diagnosing or treating patients with CNS diseases without imaging.

Imaging has established itself as an irreplaceable component of neuro-oncology, and provided much insight in all aspects of CNS tumors. Today, similar to some other medical specialties, such as bone and joint disorders, it is an integral part of the diagnosis of CNS tumors. Some pathologists, including the coauthor of this article, consider the absence of neuroimaging information almost prohibitive for accurate and realistic diagnosis in surgical neuropathology. There are numerous examples of potential pitfalls of practicing surgical neuropathology without the recognition of neuroimaging information, and the experience of expert neuropathologists suggest that it is not wise to "bet against neuroradiology." The remarkable progress in our understanding of specific entities in neuropathology also aids in a better tomorrow for patients with CNS tumors. There are encouraging developments in the attempt to classify CNS tumors with the combined help of histopathology and molecular pathology. Our recommendation for practicing surgical pathologists is that they make good friends of the neuroradiologists in their institution, because the alternative is

[a] Department of Radiology and Biomedical Imaging, UCSF School of Medicine, Room M551, 505 Parnassus Avenue, San Francisco, CA, USA; [b] Neuropathology Division, Department of Pathology, UCSF School of Medicine, UCSF Medical Center, Room M551, 505 Parnassus Avenue, San Francisco, CA 94143-0102, USA
* Corresponding author.
E-mail address: tarik.tihan@ucsf.edu

Surgical Pathology 8 (2015) 1–26
http://dx.doi.org/10.1016/j.path.2014.10.001
1875-9181/15/$ – see front matter

surgpath.theclinics.com

that pathologists achieve a good mastery of neuroradiology; a daunting task for any nonexpert.

This brief review highlights the critical elements of neuroimaging, especially of MRI, in the study and diagnosis of brain tumors, and considers some of the common entities for the diagnosis of which a good understanding of imaging characteristics is extremely helpful.

BASIC MODES AND METHODS IN NEUROIMAGING

COMPUTED TOMOGRAPHY

CT imaging was first introduced in 1972 and rapidly replaced plain films and pneumoencephalography as the tool of choice for evaluating the inside of the cranial vault. Although the earliest CT scanners with a simple X-ray tube and detector were revolutionary, they were by today's standards also incredibly slow, with the first-generation CT scanner able to image only the brain, and requiring approximately 30 minutes to image the whole brain in 13-mm-thick slices.[1] Many rapid advances in CT scanner design occurred over the subsequent decade to allow body imaging and reduce the slice time to approximately 20 seconds, with the patient moving 1 slice at a time into the scanner. In 1989, helical CT scanners were introduced, which allowed continuous motion of the patient through the CT scanner during scan acquisition, significantly improving imaging speed and image quality, and creating the opportunity for reconstruction of images in the coronal and sagittal planes. By 1998, 4-detector CT scanners were available, which allowed significantly shorter imaging time and thinner CT slices. Today, most multidetector CT (MDCT) scanners have 64 detectors, and imaging the brain may take as little as 8 seconds with a slice thickness of 0.625 mm and reconstruction of images in any desired plane without image distortion.

CT relies on simple X-ray principles, so that tissues absorbing more x-rays (generally denser tissues, such as bone) will result in a whiter image on a scan, whereas substances such as water that have very little attenuation of x-rays will result in a blacker appearance. Soft tissues, such as muscle and brain parenchyma, attenuate x-rays more than water but much less than bone, so fall in the intermediate-density appearance on CT images. To evaluate brain masses, CT exploits the subtle differences in density between normal brain parenchyma, edematous tissue, a mass, and intrinsic differences in the texture of that mass. Some tumors, such as lymphoma, tend to appear denser than brain parenchyma, whereas other tumors may have cystic low-density components like posterior fossa pilocytic astrocytomas. Similarly, some masses may have denser calcification or recent hyperdense hemorrhage. CT is the imaging tool of choice for not only detecting calcification but also for characterizing the pattern of calcification within a lesion. For example, cavernous malformations (cavernomas) are often described as having "popcorn calcification."

CONTRAST COMPUTED TOMOGRAPHY

Iodinated contrast is given intravenously and will result in a denser appearance of patent arteries and veins. Enhancement also is expected of the extraocular muscles, pituitary gland and infundibulum, and the choroid plexus. Contrast enhancement is often a helpful distinguishing feature between tumors, with, for example, the hyperenhancing nodule and prominent adjacent enhancing small blood vessels key imaging features of cerebellar hemangioblastomas. Although metastatic lesions, abscesses, and subacute infarcts and hematomas are expected to enhance, enhancement of primary brain glial neoplasms and inflammatory masses is variable and often difficult to discern on CT. Iodinated contrast can be nephrotoxic, so is not given to patients with poor renal function, and may precipitate acute renal failure. Anaphylactic reactions also are well described with iodinated contrast, and a previous allergic reaction necessitates premedication with steroids before readministration.

MRI

MRI has significantly greater sensitivity for the detection of tissue contrast enhancement. This feature, coupled with a markedly better ability to distinguish different tissues from each other (known as "contrast resolution"), makes MRI far superior to CT in the evaluation of brain tumors (**Fig. 1**). MRI has greater sensitivity for the detection of intracranial disease and, aside from the detection of calcium (and distinguishing it from blood products), is the preferred imaging modality for nearly all brain diseases.[2] In most clinical practices, the magnetic field strength is 1.5 T or 3.0 T. A higher magnetic field strength brings generally

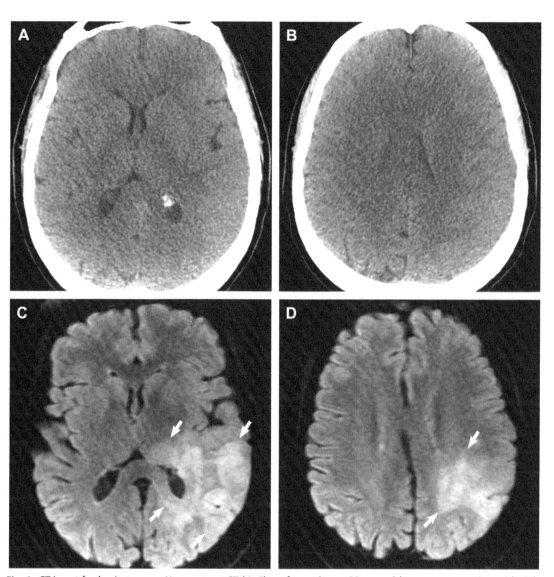

Fig. 1. CT is not for brain tumors. Noncontrast CT (*A, B*) performed on a 66-year-old woman presenting with right homonymous hemianopia. The CT is useful as a rapidly performed, readily available study to evaluate for hemorrhage, hydrocephalus, and an obvious mass. There is very subtle asymmetry but only minimal deformity of the left lateral ventricle and left sulcal effacement compared with the right side. This is best seen in retrospect after the MR was obtained. Axial FLAIR images (*C, D*) from the MRI performed later the same day show extensive infiltrating signal abnormality in the left hemisphere (*arrows*). Pathology was determined to be an anaplastic astrocytoma.

better spatial resolution, faster imaging times, and the ability to perform advanced MR techniques well.

MR images are created by first altering the direction of protons within a static magnet field through radiofrequency pulses (excitation gradients), then recording the energy emitted as they return to their lowest energy state, which is aligned in the direction of the magnet's field. Different gradient pulses are used to excite different tissues, and different tissues return to the resting state ("relax") at different rates. Imaging sequences are designed to capitalize on these relaxation characteristics as they differentiate tissues. The most frequently used brain imaging sequences are T1-weighted, T2-weighted, fluid-attenuated inversion recovery (FLAIR), and diffusion-weighted sequences (Fig. 2).

- On *T1-weighted images*, cerebrospinal fluid (CSF) and all waterlike substances are dark, fat is bright (for example, in the orbits), and white matter is subtly brighter than cortex.
- On *T2-weighted images*, "water" is bright, fat is intermediate to bright, and white matter is brighter than cortex. Most pathologic processes tend to be a little brighter than normal tissue, especially if they have edema associated with them.
- *FLAIR* sequences look like T2-weighted sequences but with the CSF (water) made black. This improves conspicuity of lesions around the ventricle margins in particular, and allows detection of abnormal substances (such as hemorrhage, pus, inflammatory debris) in CSF.
- Hemorrhage or calcifications are most readily identified on *gradient echo (GRE)* or *susceptibility-weighted (SWI)* sequences. These sequences exploit the tendency for calcifications and blood breakdown products to distort the local magnetic field, resulting in marked loss of signal. These sequences cannot, however, distinguish calcification, such as within an oligodendroglioma, from blood products due to previous hemorrhage, which we typically can do with CT.
- *Diffusion-weighted imaging (DWI)* is a rapidly acquired sequence that evaluates molecular motion and specifically the reduced ability of molecules to move (diffuse) in certain conditions. Bright signal on a DWI image, with corresponding low signal on the attenuation diffusion coefficient (ADC) image is interpreted as restriction of water motion, or "restricted diffusion." This is an expected finding in the first 7 to 10 days after a stroke when extracellular water motion is diminished because of cellular swelling with cytotoxic edema. Restricted diffusion (high DWI, low ADC) also is a feature of abscesses and of tumors with a high nuclear:cytoplasmic ratio, for example CNS lymphomas, epidermoid cysts, some metastases, and some glioblastoma multiforme (GBM). In contrast to this, facilitated diffusion (high ADC) is seen with arachnoid cysts, cysts, necrotic portion of tumors, and low-grade tumors.

CONTRAST MEDIUM CONSIDERATIONS AND CONTRAINDICATIONS

Gadolinium chelates are used for contrast enhancement and in the CNS, similar to CT,

gadolinium is given to exploit tumoral disruption of the blood-brain barrier (BBB). MR, however, is markedly more sensitive to contrast enhancement than is CT, so that some lesions that appear to have no or minimal enhancement on CT will appear readily enhancing on MRI. Gadolinium cannot be given to patients who will have impaired excretion (such as pregnant patients and patients with severe renal disease and EGFR <30), as prolonged circulation of the gadolinium contrast in the body or the fetal amniotic fluid will result in dissociation of the gadolinium ion from its chelating agent. This ion is toxic and is responsible for nephrogenic systemic fibrosis. Allergic or anaphylactic reactions are extremely rare for gadolinium chelates.

ADVANCED MRI TECHNIQUES FOR NEUROIMAGING

Although routine MRI sequences, such as T1, T2, and FLAIR, offer greater anatomic detail of brain tumors as compared with CT, the advanced MRI techniques, such as spectroscopy (MRS), perfusion, and diffusion, supply functional information about tumors. These advanced MRI techniques provide physiologic and metabolic data that reflect changes in tumor vascularity, cellularity, and proliferation. In this way, a greater contribution can be made by imaging not just in tumor diagnosis but also in characterization of malignant potential, treatment planning, and assessment of response to therapy.[3,4] Additionally, although contrast enhancement indicates the area for biopsy with BBB disruption, diffusion and perfusion may guide the surgeon to the most vascular and most cellular areas of the tumor. The area of greatest vascularity may lie in a nonenhancing portion of the tumor.[5]

MAGNETIC RESONANCE SPECTROSCOPY

MRS is the quantification within a small volume of imaged tissue of specific metabolites, such as N-acetyl aspartate (NAA), choline, creatine, and lactate. High-grade glioma typically has a high choline:creatine ratio (>2) and absent or low NAA levels. Lipid and lactate peaks also may be present. This pattern, however, is not specific for gliomas and can be seen with different pathologies. Low-grade gliomas may have a preserved MR spectrum, although myoinositol may be detected. Different MR sequences can be used to acquire this information, and although there are some technical difficulties with performing these studies, acquiring information tends to be more accurate at higher magnetic field strengths. The most frequent clinical use of MRS for brain tumor imaging is in

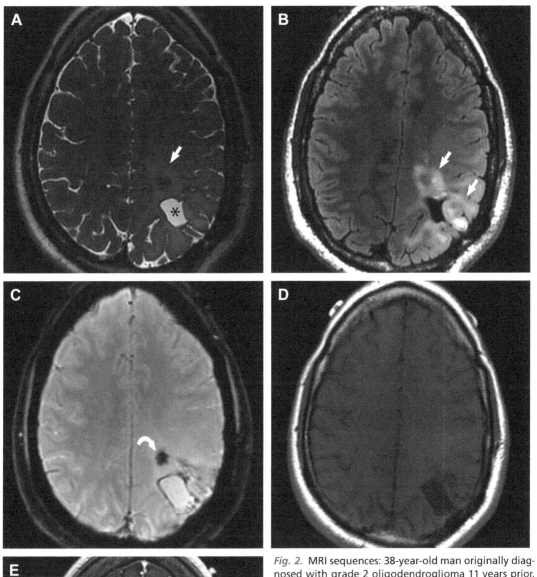

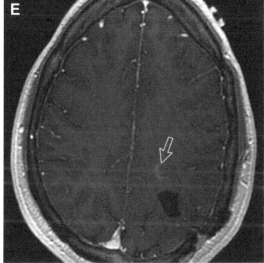

Fig. 2. MRI sequences: 38-year-old man originally diagnosed with grade 2 oligodendroglioma 11 years prior, with resection of recurrence 2 years prior shown to be grade 2 oligodendroglioma (1p/19q deleted), now presents for re-resection of recurrent disease. Axial images (*A–G*) show the routine imaging sequences used for evaluation of every brain tumor at our institution. (*A*) T2-weighted MR with bright signal intensity of CSF demonstrates a left parietal resection cavity (*asterisk*) with high signal intensity of the surrounding parenchyma indicating residual infiltrating tumor (*arrow*). This is perhaps better appreciated on (*B*), showing FLAIR sequence where CSF signal is suppressed. SWI (*C*) reveals loss of signal along the periphery of the prior resection cavity representing blood products from previous surgery. More focal rounded low signal at the deep aspect of the resection margin is blood products or calcification within recurrent tumor (*curved arrow*). Axial T1 (*D*) and postcontrast T1 (*E*) images show minimal low signal of the infiltrating component and subtle enhancement at the deep aspect (*open arrow*).

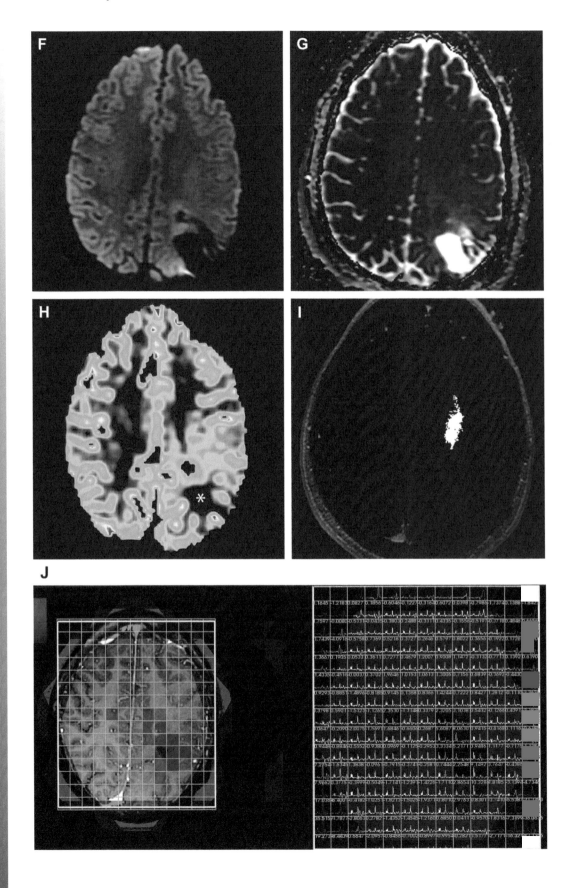

distinguishing radiation necrosis (all metabolites reduced, may have lactate/lipid peaks) from progressive GBM.[3,6]

MAGNETIC RESONANCE PERFUSION

MR perfusion aims to differentiate brain masses by determining the relative cerebral blood volume (rCBV) within a mass (relative to normal tissue), because metastases and higher-grade primary tumors tend to have elevated rCBV, correlating with vascular hyperplasia. MR perfusion with contrast administration also can estimate the permeability of the BBB, and differentiate extra-axial and nonglial tumors (such as meningiomas and metastases), which are not part of the BBB, from high-grade gliomas that have an impaired but present BBB. MR perfusion for evaluation of brain tumors with gadolinium administration can be done as contrast-enhanced or susceptibility-weighted contrast-enhanced techniques.[7]

MAGNETIC RESONANCE TRACTOGRAPHY

MR tractography (also known as diffusion tensor imaging, or DTI), uses the principle of directionality of molecular motion along nerve fibers rather than across the myelin membrane, to determine the most likely location of white matter fiber tracts. This information is then used for preoperative brain tumor planning to determine the best direction of access for biopsy and/or resection.[8]

MAGNETIC RESONANCE CONSIDERATIONS AND CONTRAINDICATIONS

MR is contraindicated if a patient has implanted hardware that is not MR compatible, such as most pacemakers, most cochlear implants, many implanted stimulators, and many aneurysm clips before 1990. Claustrophobia can be problematic for some patients in the MR scanner, although oral anxiolytics can ameliorate this problem. In the most severe claustrophobia cases and for most pediatric brain tumor imaging, general anesthesia is required. Teens and children from the age of approximately 11 are often able to remain still in the magnet with the use of MR-compatible movie goggles and relaxation techniques.

GLIAL TUMORS IN ADULTS

Gliomas are the most common primary intra-axial neoplasms of the CNS, and unfortunately, most such tumors are infiltrative and highly aggressive in the adult population. The most critical issue for gliomas is to recognize whether they belong to the class of "infiltrating" tumors that are typically relentless and progress to high-grade malignancies over time. The issue of infiltration can be difficult to interpret in small biopsies or markedly distorted specimens, and neuroimaging can suggest whether the tumor should be considered frankly infiltrating. The typical characteristics of common glial tumors in adults are summarized in the following sections.

DIFFUSE ASTROCYTOMA

Diffuse astrocytoma is a neoplasm that typically involves the deep white matter as well as the cortex, and is pathologically considered a low grade, that is, World Health Organization (WHO) grade II. Recent molecular pathologic advances identified typical genetic alterations in these tumors, which include mutations of the *IDH-1* gene, *TP53* gene, and the *ATRX* gene, which constitutes the molecular astrocytoma genotype. The only cytologic feature in these tumors is the irregularity and pleomorphism of the nuclei. The cellularity of the tissue may be only slightly altered, which can make diffuse astrocytomas extremely subtle on imaging. These predominantly supratentorial

---

Fig. 2. (*continued*). MRI sequences: 38-year-old man originally diagnosed with grade 2 oligodendroglioma 11 years prior, with resection of recurrence 2 years prior shown to be grade 2 oligodendroglioma (1p/19q deleted), now presents for re-resection of recurrent disease. Axial DWI (*F*) and the corresponding ADC (*G*) map reveal no restricted diffusion. True restricted diffusion is bright on DWI and low signal on ADC. Images (*H–J*) are advanced MRI sequences. At our institution, perfusion MR is used on nearly every tumor MR examination, DTI is used on nearly every preoperative case, and multivoxel MRS is frequently used in new tumors or treated tumors with suspected recurrence. Axial perfusion color map (*H*) demonstrates reduced rCBV at the site of cystic encephalomalacia, displayed as black color (*asterisk*), and no elevated rCBV in the area of concern, which would be demonstrated as more red or yellow in color. Note that cortex blood volume is displayed in green, and has greater blood volume than white matter displayed in blue. DTI (*I*) shows the descending corticospinal (motor) tracts are localized to white matter anterior to the MR-visible deep margin of this infiltrating tumor. Multivoxel MRS (*J*) is shown with the voxel locations overlaid on the FLAIR image on the left, and with abnormal spectra voxels highlighted on the right. There are markedly elevated choline:creatine ratios and reduced NAA (*red voxels*), suggesting tumor sites.

hemispheric tumors are generally evident as ill-defined areas of increased signal intensity on T2-weighted images, often with only subtle increase in fullness (that is, mild mass effect) and little or no surrounding edema (**Fig. 3**). Blood products are not typically evident on SWI/GRE, and calcifications are uncommon. Contrast enhancement is rarely seen with these low-grade gliomas, and should the pathology at biopsy of an enhancing lesion suggest grade II astrocytoma, concern should be raised that the highest-grade component was not sampled, as enhancement is more frequently seen with grade III, anaplastic astrocytoma.[9] Similarly, edema is more frequently a feature of higher-grade tumors. MR perfusion may show no significantly elevated

rCBV and is not generally a helpful imaging tool. Similarly MRS may not show significant alteration of metabolite ratios (specifically normal NAA, choline, and creatine).

Extensive infiltration of large portions of the brain may occur with grade II or III astrocytoma, and when there is infiltration of at least 3 lobes, it is termed gliomatosis cerebri radiologically.[10] This can be very subtle on imaging, with minimal mass effect, slightly increased T2 signal intensity, and minimal or no contrast enhancement. It may be mistaken for diffuse white matter disease, demyelinating disease, or even missed entirely. MR perfusion may be normal, and most often when it is a low-grade tumor, but an elevated rCBV suggests higher-grade tumor.[11] MRS may reveal elevated

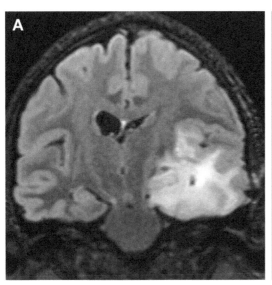

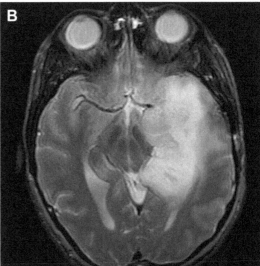

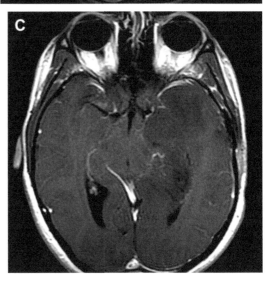

Fig. 3. Diffuse astrocytoma. Coronal FLAIR (*A*) and axial T2 (*B*) in a 33-year-old woman with many months of recurrent transient speech difficulty, confusion, and poor memory, and now presenting with a seizure, shows diffusely infiltrating FLAIR and T2 hyperintense mass in the left temporal lobe and hippocampus, extending to the insula. There is mass effect with uncal herniation. Postcontrast T1 MR (*C*) demonstrates the tumor to be of low signal intensity and without enhancement. Biopsy revealed grade 2 astrocytoma, IDH1 mutated.

choline:creatine ratio and reduced NAA, aiding in the diagnosis of subtle cases (**Fig. 4**).

OLIGODENDROGLIOMA

This diffuse, infiltrating glioma that is typical for the adult population has a classic histologic appearance that includes "fried-egg" cells, "chicken-wire" vascular pattern, and secondary structures that include conglomeration of the tumor cells around neurons, vessels, and subpial areas. The current molecular signature for oligodendroglioma includes mutation of IDH-1 or IDH-2, and the combined deletions of chromosomes 1p and 19q following a balanced translocation and loss of the derivative chromosome (ref). The oligodendroglioma is typically considered a "cortically based" tumor with multiple calcifications. These 2 features are often helpful characteristics found on imaging for suggesting the diagnosis of oligodendroglioma. Another helpful feature is the location, with most oligodendrogliomas being in the frontal and temporal lobes. Oligodendrogliomas tend to appear well-defined, have low signal on T1, and are heterogeneously hyperintense on T2-weighted images with little or no surrounding vasogenic edema. Tumor calcifications can be suggested low signal intensity on T1-weighted and T2-weighted MR images, and with loss of signal with SWI/GRE sequences. MR cannot distinguish calcification from hemorrhage but CT will readily identify the high-density coarse calcifications (**Fig. 5**).[12] The tumors with 1p/19q deletions were suggested to have more calcifications and ill-defined margins.[13] In distinction to low-grade diffuse astrocytomas, contrast enhancement is common in low-grade oligodendrogliomas, and they are seen in approximately 50% of cases. The enhancoomont ic usually mild and more often much less than that in grade III tumors and mixed oligoastrocytomas. Both grade II and grade III oligodendrogliomas may have an elevated rCBV on MR perfusion, with a tendency for greater rCBV with the higher-grade tumors.[14]

GLIOBLASTOMAS

The most common glial tumor type among the adult population is the glioblastoma that demonstrates all the histologic features of a highly malignant neoplasm. The typical tumor is a markedly pleomorphic neoplasm with vascular endothelial proliferation and necrosis. The 2 variants for glioblastomas, the giant cell glioblastoma and the gliosarcoma, tend to be more superficially located, often associated with dura mater, and appear more circumscribed. The gliosarcoma also has a tendency to demonstrate leptomeningeal spread and occasionally divergent differentiation that includes chondromatous and even osseous components. Additional subtypes that are not considered as unique variants in the WHO classification are the small-cell glioblastoma and glioblastoma with primitive neuroectodermal tumor–like component. A controversial entity, glioblastoma with oligodendroglial component also has been described.

The molecular pathology of glioblastomas is far more complex, and attempts to group these tumors based on the molecular expression patterns have been at best tenuous. Recent studies suggested 5-tiered or 4-tiered molecular subgroups, but with the exception of the so-called mesenchymal subgroup, these analyses have been unsuccessful in predicting distinct clinicopathological categories. Recent studies also suggested that these molecular subgroups may reflect the tumor composition and sampling bias rather than true genetic categories.

Earlier studies on glioblastomas have uncovered at least 2 genetically distinct groups that are associated with specific clinical features.[15] The best-defined groups are the primary or "de novo" glioblastoma and the secondary glioblastoma.[16]

- Primary or de novo glioblastoma has been reported in the older populations, with a relatively rapid onset of symptoms, no evidence of a previous low-grade neoplasm, and genetic alterations in the *EGFR* gene, PI3K pathways, including *PTEN* losses. This type constitutes the greater majority of glioblastomas in most studies.
- Secondary glioblastoma, on the other hand, often progresses from a lower-grade infiltrating glioma, occurs in a younger age group, has a longer symptomatic period, and is often associated with *IDH-1 TP53* gene mutations as well as *ATRX* mutations.[17]

The molecular alterations for most cases in each group are mutually exclusive (ie, finding *EGFR* amplification would often suggest absence of *IDH-1* mutation in a particular glioblastoma).[18] There are, however, tumors that do not fit into the typical primary and secondary glioblastoma definitions. Further studies are needed to generate a more precise histopathologic/molecular grouping of glioblastomas, but these studies suggest that glioblastomas constitute a spectrum of neoplasms with distinct histologic and genetic characteristics, and are by no means a pure diagnostic category.

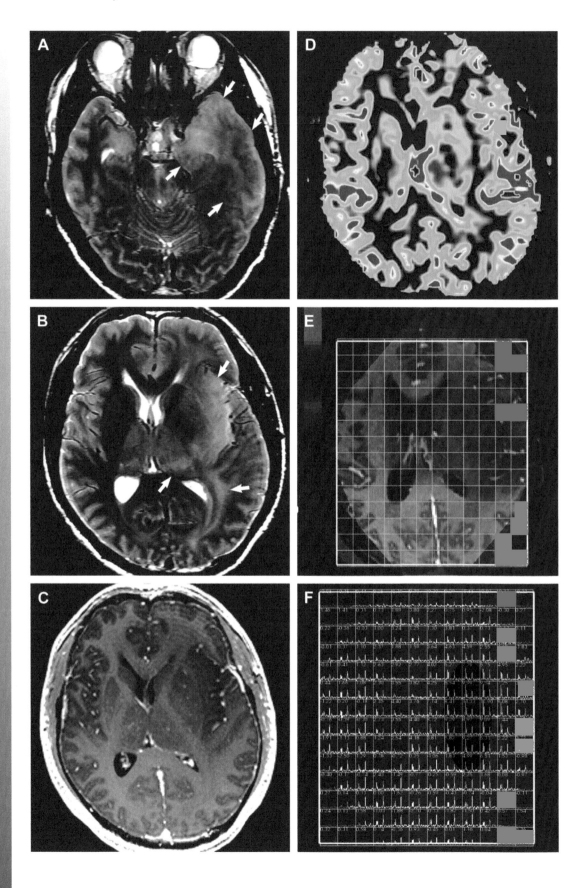

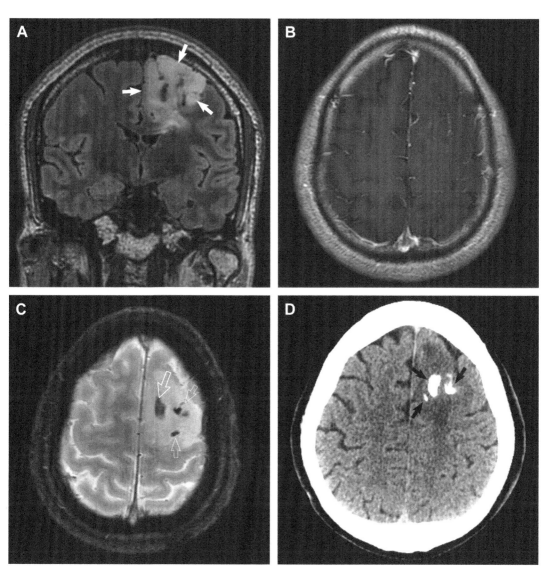

Fig. 5. Oligodendroglioma/oligoastrocytoma: 57-year-old man, previously well and presenting with first-time gener-alized tonic-clonic seizure. Coronal FLAIR (*A*) shows a heterogeneous mass involving the left superior and middle frontal gyri. Note that there is involvement with thickening and high signal of both the cortex and white matter (*white arrows*). Axial postcontrast T1 (*B*) shows no abnormal enhancement, but SWI (*C*) reveals focal wedges of mark-edly low signal intensity (*open arrows*), suggesting blood products or calcification. Axial noncontrast CT (*D*) deter-mines these areas to be coarse calcifications (*black arrows*). The frontal location, cortical involvement, and calcifications suggest oligodendroglial neoplasm. Subtotal resection revealed grade 2 oligodendroglial tumor, 1p/19q deleted, *IDH-1* mutation, p53 negative.

Fig. 4. Gliomatosis cerebri: 40-year-old man with several weeks of lethargy and diplopia. Axial T2 MR (*A, B*) shows asymmetric hyperintensity and expansion of the left temporal lobe, with signal extending into the left insula and occipital lobe along white matter fiber tracts (*arrows*). Postcontrast T1 MR (*C*) shows no abnormal enhancement. Note more subtle involvement of the left thalamus and spread to the right thalamus and right temporal lobe. MR perfusion color map (*D*) shows no increased rCBV. Multivoxel MRS (*E, F*), however, reveals markedly abnormal metabolite ratios in the left insula and thalamus (*red ellipse*) with elevated choline: creatine and low NAA. This imaging pattern is highly suggestive of low-grade infiltrating astrocytoma.

Imaging Findings in Glioblastoma

Just as the pathology demonstrates necrosis and vascular proliferation, the imaging findings typically reflect this with a heterogeneous appearance on T1, T2, and FLAIR sequences, and contrast enhancement. Susceptibility images (SWI) frequently show areas of microhemorrhage manifest as multiple punctate foci of signal loss, and acute intratumoral hemorrhage may be a feature of presentation of these aggressive grade IV gliomas, although this is uncommon (Fig. 6).[19,20]

Areas of necrosis are typically low signal on T1 and high signal on T2 and have an irregular, variably thick enhancing rim (Figs. 7 and 8). GBMs frequently have surrounding T2 hyperintense vasogenic edema, but it is not possible by imaging to differentiate edema alone from tumor infiltration, and we expect that the extent of tumor is greater than what is evident on T2 or contrast-enhanced imaging. Other than ring enhancement, it is not uncommon to find solid, nodular, or patchy areas of tumoral enhancement within GBMs.[21]

DWI may show focal areas of restricted diffusion with high signal on DWI and low signal on ADC. These foci often correspond with solid regions of enhancement and show elevated rCBV on perfusion MR. Any of these 3 features (restricted diffusion, solid enhancement, and elevated rCBV) suggest high-grade foci that should be considered as targets for biopsy (3,5).

GLIAL TUMORS IN CHILDREN

Pediatric gliomas are a heterogeneous group of neoplasms that range from circumscribed and low grade to highly infiltrative and malignant. There is increasing recognition that gliomas in the pediatric population are quite distinct from their adult counterparts, even when the name of the neoplasm suggests otherwise. Unlike the adult gliomas, the overwhelming majority of pediatric gliomas occur in the posterior fossa, with mostly solid or solid/cystic architecture and are low grade. High-grade gliomas and oligodendroglial tumors are rare in the pediatric age group.

PILOCYTIC ASTROCYTOMAS

The most common pediatric glioma is the pilocytic astrocytoma (PA) that can occur anywhere in the CNS but has a propensity to involve the posterior fossa and the optic system. The tumor is also associated with neurofibromatosis 1 (NF1). The histology of the typical PA is that of a biphasic, compact glial neoplasm with bipolar, "hairlike" glial cells, Rosenthal fibers, and eosinophilic granular bodies. The histologic variation among PAs is remarkable and some examples may not be readily diagnosed as such. Specifically, oligodendrogliomalike and polar spongioblastomalike patterns have been challenging in the past.

Recent studies on PAs have uncovered significant advances on the molecular characteristics of this neoplasm, and the reader is referred to the article by Reis and colleagues, elsewhere in this issue, for a more detailed discussion of molecular features of PA.

Imaging Findings in Pilocytic Astrocytomas

PAs tend to have reliably predictable findings on imaging. In the posterior fossa, they typically arise in the cerebellar hemisphere with an eccentric enhancing nodule in association with a nonenhancing, or peripherally enhancing cyst. The cyst typically compresses the fourth ventricle and often results in hydrocephalus with third and lateral ventricular enlargement (Fig. 9). Less commonly, PA appears as a more solid, heterogeneously enhancing lateral cerebellar mass. Calcifications and hemorrhage are not typical imaging features with either imaging presentation.[22,23] With DWI sequences, the solid part of the lesion will show only mildly restricted diffusion, which can be an additional differentiating feature from other posterior fossa pediatric neoplasms, such as medulloblastoma and ependymoma.[24] There are, however, additional imaging features to differentiate these neoplasms from PA. Medulloblastoma is most often a midline solid mass within the posterior fossa, and the patients are typically younger in age (2–6 years) than PA. In the posterior fossa, ependymomas arise in the fourth ventricle and extend through the foramina to the cerebellopontine angle. Calcification is not uncommon and enhancement may be minimal to moderate but is typically heterogeneous.

PAs are also found in association with the optic nerves/chiasm/optic tract, and this is the more frequent location in patients with NF1.[25] These tumors are typically solid, T2 hyperintense, and extend along these pathways, expanding the white matter tracts and are associated with enhancement. Enhancement is a typical finding of PA and can be misleading to radiologists, as enhancement is often a feature of high-grade neoplasms.

DIFFUSE ASTROCYTOMA AND GLIOBLASTOMA

Diffuse astrocytic tumors and their most malignant form, glioblastoma, present a unique clinical and molecular character among children. It is clear

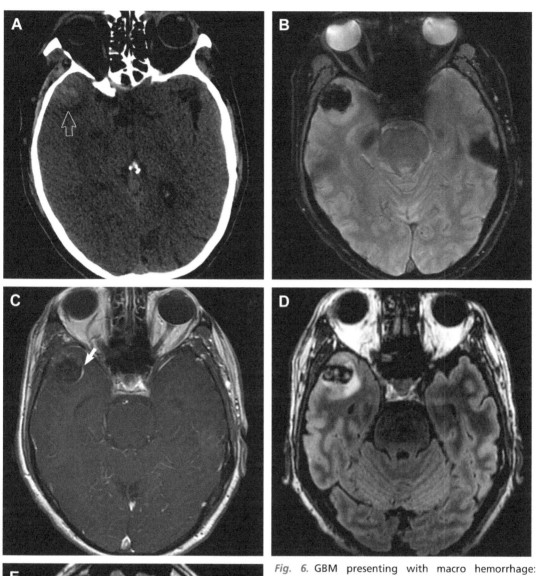

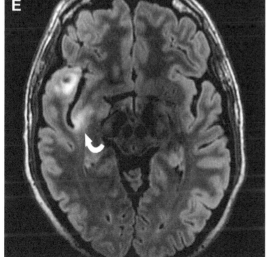

Fig. 6. GBM presenting with macro hemorrhage: 54-year-old man presented with a first-time seizure. CT scan in the emergency room (*A*) showed a subtle right anterior temporal lobe mass, interpreted as recent hemorrhage (*open arrow*). One of the prime considerations for this appearance was a hemorrhagic cavernous malformation. MRI was then performed. Axial SWI (*B*) shows marked loss of signal intensity in keeping with the interpretation of hemorrhage. Post-contrast T1 (*C*) demonstrates only subtle curvilinear enhancement at the medial aspect of the hemorrhage (*white arrow*). Axial FLAIR (*D, E*), however, revealed not only a little high signal around the periphery of the hemorrhage, as might be seen with an acute hemorrhage, but also infiltrating signal in the posterior aspect of the right insula (*curved arrow*), which should not be found with a cavernous malformation. This raised concern for an underlying infiltrating neoplasm. Surgical resection revealed glioblastoma multiforme.

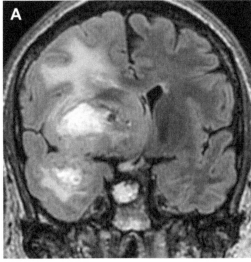

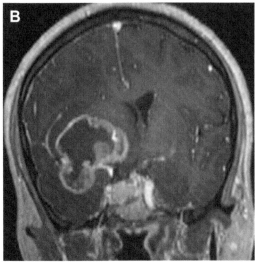

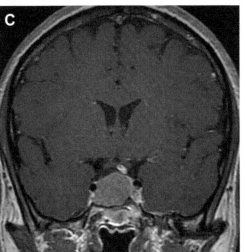

Fig. 7. Primary GBM: 58-year-old man with increasing headaches, subtle left-sided weakness, and recent trans-sphenoidal surgery for a pituitary macroadenoma. Coronal FLAIR (*A*) and postcontrast T1 MR (*B*) demonstrate extensive infiltrative FLAIR hyperintensity in the right temporal lobe, insula, and inferior frontal lobe with rim enhancement of the heterogeneous tumor. There is marked mass effect. (*C*) Coronal postcontrast T1 image from the brain MRI performed almost 6 months prior when the patient was diagnosed with a pituitary macroadenoma. The remaining brain MRI appears normal even in retrospect.

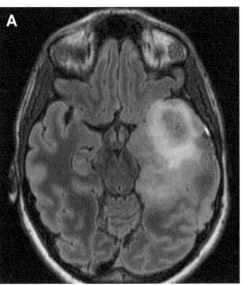

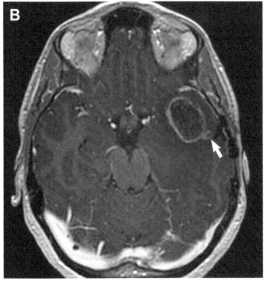

Fig. 8. Secondary GBM: 35-year-old woman imaged 18 months after diagnosis of grade 2 astrocytoma and commencement of temozolomide therapy (this is the same patient as Fig. 3). Axial FLAIR (*A*) and postcontrast T1 MR (*B*) show in addition to the diffusely expanded temporal lobe, a more focal large heterogeneous left anterior temporal lobe mass with rim enhancement, and an adjacent smaller rim-enhancing nodule (*arrow*). Rebiopsy and subtotal resection revealed glioblastoma multiforme (p53 positive, EGFR negative, PTEN negative, positive for methylated MGMT).

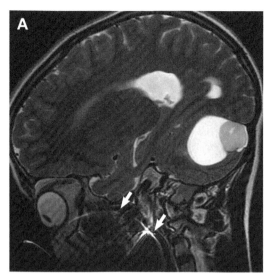

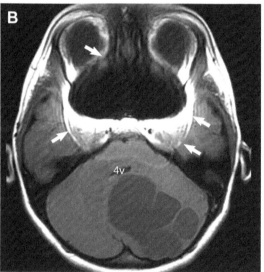

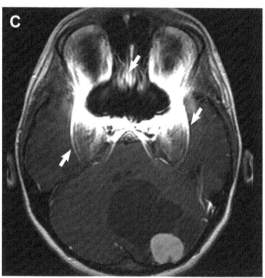

Fig. 9. PA: 12-year-old girl presenting with dizziness and vertigo. Sagittal T2-weighted MR (*A*) and axial T1 (*B*) demonstrate a mass in the left cerebellar hemisphere, extending to the midline and deforming the fourth ventricle (4v). The mass is predominantly cystic with high T2 signal similar to CSF, but T1 signal slightly brighter than CSF. Axial postcontrast T1 MR (*C*) reveals a 2 × 2-cm intensely enhancing nodule at the posterior margin of the mass. This appearance is highly suggestive of a grade 1 PA, which it proved to be at resection. Note the extensive artifact (*arrows*) on all 3 sequences, but especially the T1 precontrast and postcontrast images, from the patient's dental braces, which distort the local magnetic field.

that the driver mutations and molecular alterations are quite distinct between adult and pediatric diffuse gliomas. Two specific groups among the pediatric population are the diffuse intrinsic pontine glioma (DIPG) and the bithalamic astrocytoma, both of which are infiltrating and aggressive neoplasms. Although these tumors are also graded in the same fashion as the adult counterparts, it is clear that such grading grossly underestimates the aggressive nature of most of these tumors. A review of the molecular characteristics of these tumors is presented by Pekmezci and colleagues, elsewhere in this issue.

By definition, DIPG is found in the pons and brainstem, and on presentation typically have an expansile, T2/FLAIR hyperintense infiltrative appearance with ill-defined margins. These tumors tend to obstruct the fourth ventricle, resulting in hydrocephalus and may appear to engulf the basilar artery. Contrast enhancement is variable within these tumors, but ring enhancement at the time of diagnosis is a predictor of poorer survival (**Fig. 10**).[26] Overall, DIPG has a poor prognosis, with little response to chemotherapy regimens, and radiation is the mainstay of therapy.[27] Radiologists are investigating advanced MRI techniques to try to determine features that might stratify DIPG into subgroups with better and poorer survival. Using DWI, lower ADC values, which often correlate with greater cellularity, appear to predict a poorer prognosis.[28] Perfusion MRI suggests that, as with other (non-PA) brain tumors, areas with higher rCBV suggest tumor angiogenesis and indicate more aggressive tumors.[29]

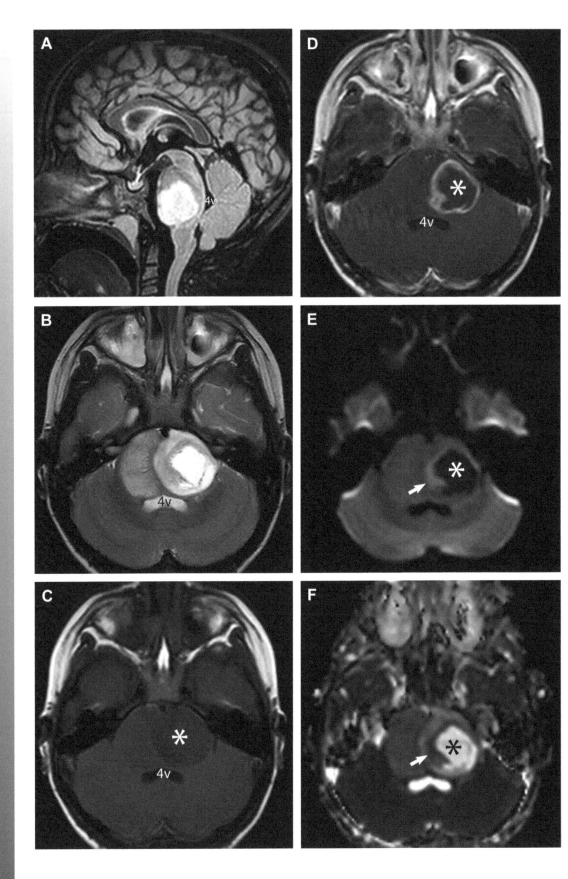

Pediatric thalamic gliomas clinically and prognostically appear to be similar to DIPG, generally being of high grade and having a poor outcome.[30] On imaging, expansion and T2/FLAIR hyperintensity of the thalamus is expected with ill-defined margins more often a feature of higher-grade tumors. Enhancement is variable, and although low-grade infiltrating astrocytomas do not typically have enhancement, moderate enhancement is commonly seen with PAs (Fig. 11). Of the low-grade thalamic tumors, bithalamic involvement is a predictor of reduced progressive free and overall survival, so careful evaluation for contralateral disease is important on MRI.[31]

MENINGIOMAS

Meningiomas are the most common extra-axial tumors primary to the CNS, and their clinicopathological characteristics are well described. The current classification scheme used by WHO provides an independent prognostic feature with the typing and grading of meningiomas. Based on this scheme, atypical or WHO grade II meningiomas have a higher rate of local recurrence that the typical grade I meningioma, whereas grade III meningiomas are highly aggressive and lethal. The overwhelming majority of meningiomas are grade I neoplasms, and gross total resection leads to cure in most cases. Some variants, namely the clear cell, chordoid, papillary, and rhabdoid meningiomas are more aggressive tumors and are considered to be higher grade regardless of other histologic features. In addition, brain parenchymal invasion appears to be a sign of a more aggressive meningioma, and the presence of this histologic feature implies at least a WHO grade II neoplasm.

Typical markers helpful for the diagnosis of meningiomas include epithelial membrane antigen (EMA) and somatostatin receptor 2A (SSTR2A), which are positive in the overwhelming majority of tumors. Most meningiomas also express varying levels of progresteron receptors.

The molecular pathology of meningiomas is being revealed in recent studies, and in addition to its association with neurofibromatosis 2, multiple meningiomas also have been associated with additional genetic alterations.[32] Recent studies have found Chr 22 loss as the most common alteration, but also reported mutations in TRAF7, AKT1, KLF4, and SMO genes.[33]

Most meningiomas occur in the supratentorial brain with nearly half of these involving the dura of the convexities or falx. The remaining lesions have a predilection for the greater sphenoid wing, the olfactory groove of the anterior cranial fossa, and the parasellar region. Infratentorially, the cerebellopontine angle is the most frequent location. Fewer than 5% involve the optic nerve sheath and the pineal region (so-called falcotentorial meningiomas), or occur within the ventricles or within skull base bones as intraosseous meningiomas.[21]

IMAGING FINDINGS IN MENINGIOMAS

These extra-axial lesions are most often characterized by a clear site of dural attachment and contrast enhancement. Aside from these 2 relatively constant features, meningiomas may have a widely varying appearance on imaging, while still having grade 1 histopathology (Fig. 12). About a quarter of meningiomas will have calcification evident on CT that may be solid, diffuse, focal, coarse, "sunburst," or sandlike. The adjacent bone may appear thickened and hyperdense (interpreted as hyperostosis) or have an irregular cortical margin with prominent adjacent calvarial vascular grooves. Hyperostosis with dense thickened appearance of bone is a common imaging finding in association with the calvarium and is a helpful differentiating feature. Abnormal dilation of the sphenoid sinus can occur with planum sphenoidale/tuberculum sellae meningiomas, known as pneumosinus dilatans. This uncommon imaging finding, which can be recognized on CT or MR, is virtually pathognomonic for meningioma.

MR signal intensity is also variable, although often isointense to brain parenchyma on T1, hyperintense on T2/FLAIR, and frequently showing signal loss on SWI/GRE from calcifications. Nearly

Fig. 10. Diffuse infiltrating pontine glioma: 4-year-old boy with progressively worsening ataxia. Sagittal FLAIR (A) and axial T2 (B) and T1 (C) MR demonstrate a T2 hyperintense, T2 hypointense bilobed mass expanding the pons and deforming the fourth ventricle (4v). The pons is so expanded there is little CSF space remaining in the cerebellopontine angles. The left aspect of the pons has a more hyperintense central component, which is lower on T1 and higher in T2 signal, indicating a cystic component (asterisk). After contrast administration (D), there is complete rim enhancement of this component of the DIPG. Axial DWI (E) and the corresponding ADC image (F) show facilitated diffusion within the cystic component (asterisk) but subtle restricted diffusion in the medial thicker rim that enhances (arrow), suggesting this is the highest-grade region within the tumor.

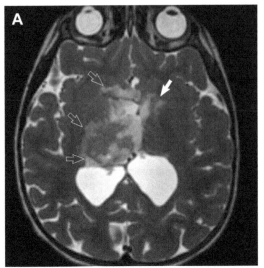

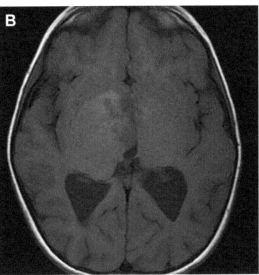

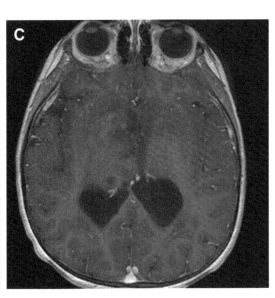

Fig. 11. Thalamic astrocytoma: 6-year-old girl presents with a possible seizure. Axial T2 (*A*) and T1 (*B*) MR shows a large heterogeneous infiltrative mass involving the right thalamus and basal ganglia (*open arrows*). There was also extensive infiltration into the medial temporal lobe and brainstem, and infiltration to the contralateral side (*arrow*). Postcontrast T1 MR (*C*) revealed no abnormal enhancement. Stereotactic biopsy of the right basal ganglia revealed a grade 2 infiltrating astrocytoma, which was negative for *BRAF* V600E mutation and *PTEN* deletion.

all meningiomas show intense enhancement with gadolinium, unless they are heavily calcified, and nearly all will reveal a dural site of attachment, often described on imaging as a "dural tail." Areas of cystic change within meningiomas may be found and rarely fat density (CT) or intensity (MRI) with the lipomatous variant.

Vasogenic edema in adjacent displaced brain parenchyma is seen as irregularly contoured high T2 signal around the lesion, which is not restricted on DWI. The degree of edema associated with meningiomas is highly variable and does not predict tumor grade. Clear evidence of parenchymal invasion, however, or lytic destruction of bone suggests atypical or malignant meningioma, or an alternative pathologic diagnosis for a dura-based mass, such as metastasis, lymphoma, or hemangiopericytoma.

Advanced MR techniques, such as MRS and MR perfusion, show altered metabolites and elevated rCBV, respectively, within meningioma, but do not distinguish typical from atypical and malignant entities. MRS is often technically difficult to perform next to the skull bone and scalp fat, which result in artifacts, and tumoral calcification makes both MRS and MR perfusion technically challenging because of susceptibility artifacts.[34,35] Generally, however, atypical or malignant meningiomas tend to have higher rCBV than grade I meningiomas.

METASTASES IN CENTRAL NERVOUS SYSTEM TUMORS

Metastatic tumors in the CNS are often a consideration for lesions in the adult population, and

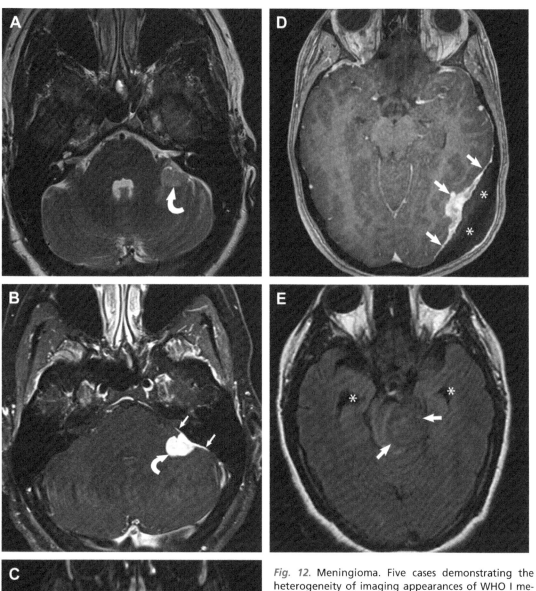

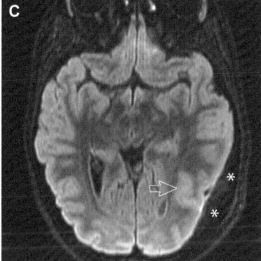

Fig. 12. Meningioma. Five cases demonstrating the heterogeneity of imaging appearances of WHO I meningiomas, and some of the commonalities. (*A, B*) Axial T2 (*A*) and postcontrast T1 (*B*) MR in a 52-year-old woman demonstrates a posterior fossa mass (*curved arrow*) that is only subtly hyperintense to cerebellum, and is associated with a tiny amount of edema, but intense enhancement. There is a dural attachment along the posterior face of the petrous temporal bone with anterior and posterior "dural tails" (*arrows*). These are not seen with schwannomas. (*C, D*) Axial FLAIR (*C*) and postcontrast T1 (*D*) in a 30-year-old woman with chronic migraines shows asymmetry of the occipital calvarium (*asterisks*) and subtle increase in brain FLAIR signal (*open arrow*). Hyperostosis is manifest as low signal on all sequences. (*E, F*) Axial FLAIR (*E*) and postcontrast T1 (*F*) MR in a 29-year-old woman with headaches reveals a mass (*arrows*) isointense to brain but intensely although heterogeneously enhancing, and attached to the petroclival region. The mass compresses the midbrain and results in hydrocephalus with dilated temporal horns (*asterisks*), although is not associated with parenchymal edema.

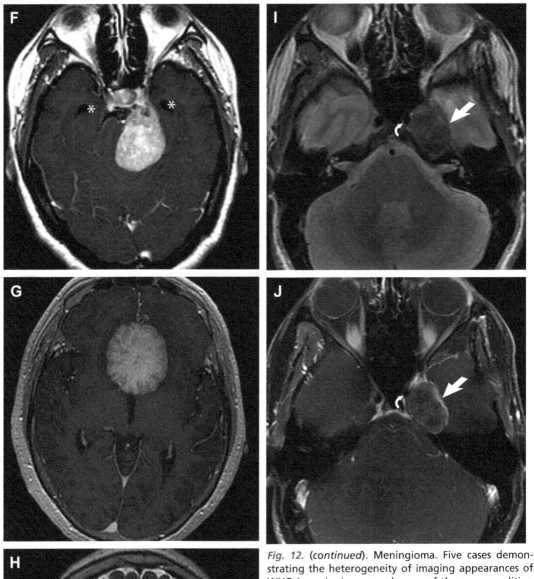

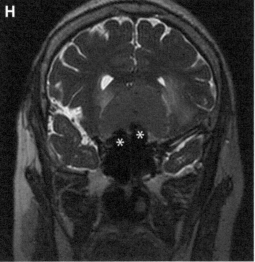

Fig. 12. (*continued*). Meningioma. Five cases demonstrating the heterogeneity of imaging appearances of WHO I meningiomas, and some of the commonalities. (*G, H*) Axial T1 postcontrast (*G*) and coronal T2 (*H*) demonstrate a midline intensely enhancing mass isointense to brain on T2, centered on the planum sphenoidale. Note ballooning of the sphenoid sinuses (*asterisks*) above the floor of the anterior cranial fossa. This is known as pneumosinus dilatans and is highly suggestive of meningioma. (*I, J*) Axial T2 (*I*) and postcontrast T1 (*J*) demonstrate a mass (*arrow*) in the left middle cranial fossa associated with the cavernous sinus and displacing the cavernous internal carotid artery (*curved arrow*). The mass is only mildly enhancing and is very low on T2 signal. This is compatible with extensive calcifications and the biopsy finding of psammomatous meningioma.

constitute the most common neoplastic process in the CNS. Although most metastatic lesions, especially those with multiple foci, do not come to the attention of pathologists, the sheer number of patients with CNS metastases make this group one of the most common lesions encountered in the brain and spinal cord. Histologically, the metastatic lesions can demonstrate the cytologic and morphologic features of the primary organ or may be too poorly differentiated to be readily recognized. Clinical knowledge of a malignant tumor elsewhere in the body, especially presence of metastases elsewhere, are of great help, but occasionally a primary CNS tumor can coexist with a carcinoma of a solid organ. Thus, a thorough workup and morphologic characterization with immunohistochemical workup, and rarely molecular marker analysis, can identify the origin of the metastatic tumor, especially if the origin is not known at the time of surgery. There are increasing numbers of markers that aid the pathologist in recognizing the tumor's origin, and rarely such efforts fail due to the undifferentiated nature of the malignant neoplasm. Algorithms and approach to workup of metastatic tumors have been comprehensively discussed in recent articles, and the reader is referred to these careful reports for help in the workup of such cases. However, neuroimaging studies can readily identify the neoplasm as a metastatic lesion preoperatively, making the job of the pathologist much easier.

IMAGING FINDINGS IN CENTRAL NERVOUS SYSTEM METASTASES

Metastases are evident on CT or MR as enhancing masses that may be parenchymal, dural, or leptomeningeal in location or arise from the skull base or calvarium. Postcontrast CT may detect large brain lesions, and the bone windows on CT are generally good for the detection of lytic or sclerotic bone metastases. CT is, however, relatively insensitive for the detection of cerebral metastases and MR with gadolinium is strongly recommended. MR is also better able to characterize masses than CT and differentiate abscess, metastases, and primary glial neoplasms, for example.

Although metastases can mimic a wide variety of disease on MR, one of the most useful differentiating features from primary CNS neoplasms is the presence of multiple distinct well-defined lesions, which typically are intensely enhancing. Parenchymal metastases favor the grey-white junction and most are hemispheric. Approximately 15% are found in the cerebellum, 3% in the basal ganglia, and fewer than 1% in the brainstem.[21] Metastases may be solid or cystic, and may

contain blood-fluid levels or even present as cerebral hemorrhage with the primary lesion not clearly evident. Vasogenic edema is a common association with metastases, although is variable in extent even for different lesions in the same patient and may not be evident at all (Fig. 13).

In complex or confusing cases, and particularly if only 1 brain lesion is evident, advanced imaging techniques may offer useful information to distinguish solitary metastases from enhancing (and therefore usually high-grade) primary brain tumors.[3,4]

Magnetic Resonance Perfusion

MR perfusion can be very helpful in distinguishing metastases from high-grade enhancing primary cerebral tumors. Although both lesions will have elevated rCBV from the increased vascularity, metastatic lesions will not have a preserved BBB, and so the contrast-enhanced perfusion curve will reflect the absence of a BBB, and "leakiness" of the vessels to contrast (see Fig. 13). Some GBMs with significantly impaired BBB can, however, mimic this "metastasis perfusion curve." The discovery of such outliers has led to more careful evaluation of the peritumoral region; that is, the area peripheral to the enhancing rim of the brain lesion. The nature of GBMs is to infiltrate the surrounding tissue and grow beyond the area of enhancement on imaging, whereas metastatic lesions (with or without edema) are more sharply circumscribed pathologically. If the rCBV in the peritumoral region of enhancing primary brain tumor is elevated as compared with the contralateral brain, this suggests GBM.[36]

Magnetic Resonance Spectroscopy

The MRS ratios obtained within brain lesions are often nonspecifically abnormal and therefore not helpful for distinguishing brain lesions. Again, however, the peritumoral metabolite ratios (NAA:creatine, choline:creatine, and choline:NAA) indicate that glioblastomas can be differentiated from metastases that have patterns more like normal brain. More recently, the evaluation of lipid and macromolecules within tumors using short-echo time single-voxel MRS has also suggested that GBM and solitary metastasis can be distinguished with high accuracy.[37]

Diffusion-Weighted Imaging

DWI does not usually show restriction in metastases or in primary brain tumors, except in very cellular areas of a solid tumor. The presence of restricted diffusion within a cystic, rim-enhancing lesion, however, suggests an abscess, and this can be an important preoperative observation indicating that

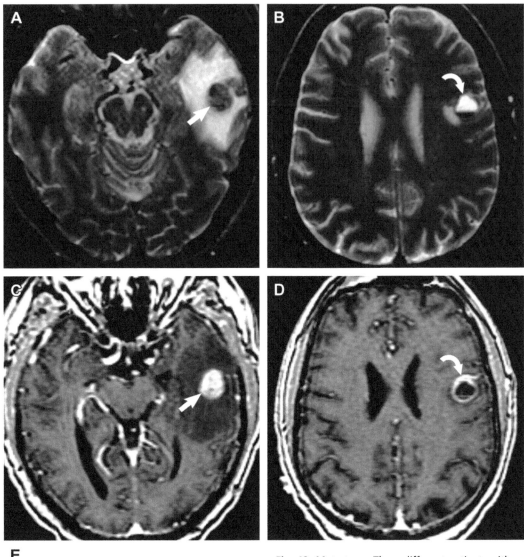

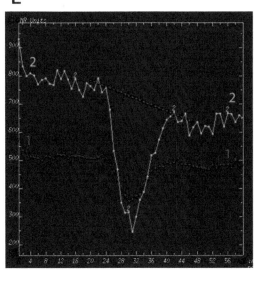

Fig. 13. Metastases. Three different patients with metastatic melanoma illustrating some distinguishing features and behaviors of metastases. (*A–E*) A 63-year-old man with right shoulder melanoma resected 15 years previously, now "talking gibberish" according to his wife. Axial T2 (*A, B*) and postcontrast T1 (*C, D*) show 2 lesions. In the left temporal lobe there is a solidly enhancing round mass with extensive surrounding vasogenic edema (*arrow*). More superiorly in the left frontal lobe there is a rim-enhancing cystic mass with a blood-fluid level, and significantly less edema (*curved arrow*). Two separate well-defined lesions like this strongly suggest the diagnosis of metastases. Dynamic susceptibility-weighted contrast-enhanced MR perfusion was performed on the frontal lesion with the purple curve ("1") representing normal contralateral brain and the green curved ("2") representing the enhancing margin of the metastasis. The deeper drop in signal of the green curve indicates a greater rCBV. The curve does not return to a baseline level, which is consistent with a metastasis. A primary brain tumor would be expected to return close to the baseline curve.

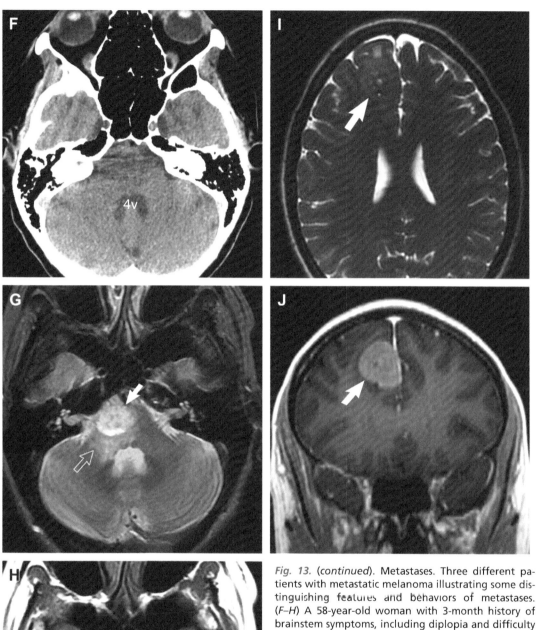

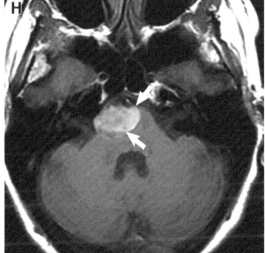

Fig. 13. (continued). Metastases. Three different patients with metastatic melanoma illustrating some distinguishing features and behaviors of metastases.
(F–H) A 58-year-old woman with 3-month history of
brainstem symptoms, including diplopia and difficulty
swallowing, and a melanoma excised from her back
2 years earlier. Axial noncontrast CT (F) shows very subtle low density of the pons, and subtle deformity of
the contour of the fourth ventricle (4v). Axial T2 MR
(G) reveals a rounded pontine mass (arrow) with
edema involving the brachium pontis (open arrow).
On T1 MR (H), there is bright signal that is intrinsic
to the mass in this noncontrast study. T1 intensity on
a noncontrast MR suggests fat, calcium, methemo-
globin (hemorrhage), or melanin. (I, J) Axial T2 (I)
and coronal postcontrast T1 (J) MR in a 29-year-old
woman with a history of metastatic melanoma. This
frontal falcine-based mass (arrow) mimics a meningioma on MR and has no significant edema and only
mild mass effect. Imaging at one time point only
cannot differentiate the 2 entities; however, the patient also had 2 other lesions in the brain parenchyma.
This was metastatic melanoma at resection.

drainage rather than resection is necessary. Evaluation on DWI of the peritumoral region, however, again appears to be helpful with the mean minimum ADC values and mean ADC ratios in the peritumoral regions of glioblastomas significantly higher than in the peritumoral region of metastases.

COMMON MIMICS OF NEOPLASIA IN NEUROIMAGING

The differential diagnosis of CNS neoplasms includes a large list of non-neoplastic entities, and this list is different for both the neuroradiologist and the pathologist (Table 1). For some entities, the diagnosis may be quite challenging in neuroimaging, whereas the histologic diagnosis is made with much ease. Obviously, the reverse is true for some other cases, in which there is much more certainty about the presence of a neoplasm on radiological grounds, but the pathologist may have substantial difficulty in reaching the same conclusion. For the purposes of this article, we focus on lesions that may resemble neoplasms on radiological

assessment. This discussion will help to understand the radiological interpretation in cases in which there is discrepancy between the radiological and pathologic diagnosis. Obviously, one of the most critical issues before embarking on the task of providing a differential diagnosis is the sample adequacy. Although neuroimaging studies can recognize the lesion(s) and their relationship with the CNS structures in every case, pathologists may see only a small, and occasionally unrepresentative, sample of the process. Therefore, the first inquiry for the pathologist before disputing the neuroimaging impression is an inquiry on sample adequacy, and neuroimaging as well as the neurosurgeon's impression are most helpful in this way. Once the sample adequacy issue is addressed, then the list of differential diagnosis can be more objectively scrutinized to reach the best interpretation of the patient's disease. A comprehensive review of CNS tumor mimics is beyond the scope of this article, but a list of mimics based on the topographic distribution of lesions can aid in the diagnosis. The reader is referred to more comprehensive reviews such as that of Bradley and Rees.[38]

Table 1
Mimickers of central nervous system tumors and features to aid in their radiological differential diagnosis

Site	Impression	Mimicker	Key Imaging Feature
Supratentorial	Glioma or metastasis	Infarct	Acute: no enhancement but restricted DWI. Subacute: Enhances, not restricted DWI. History and evolution over time are helpful.
	HGG or metastasis	Hematoma	Enhance peripherally in subacute phase. Anterior temporal or inferior frontal most often. Blood products on SWI/GRE.
	HGG	Tumefactive demyelinating lesion	Look for additional small demyelinating plaques. May be extremely difficult to distinguish.
	HGG or metastasis	Granulomatous disease	Look for other areas of abnormality, such as leptomeningeal. Often difficult for solitary lesion; may benefit from chest CT, CSF sampling.
	HGG or metastasis	Abscess	Restricted diffusion in center of lesion: low ADC. History may or may not help.
	Progressive HGG	Radionecrosis	MRS metabolites low, +/– lipid/lactate. MR perfusion variable, may be low.
	HGG	Lymphoma	Tends to have more solid enhancement. These areas often have restricted diffusion also.
	HGG, meningioma	Solitary metastasis	Contrast-enhanced MR perfusion of lesion shows absent BBB. Peritumoral perfusion, ADC and MRS normal.
Infratentorial	Meningioma	Schwannoma	No dural attachment site/no dural tail.
	Meningioma	Epidermoid	Restricted diffusion and no enhancement.

Abbreviations: ADC, apparent diffusion coefficient; BBB, blood-brain barrier; CSF, cerebrospinal fluid; CT, computed tomography; DWI, diffusion-weighted imaging; GRE, gradient recalled echo; HGG, high-grade glioma; MRS, magnetic resonance spectroscopy; SWI, susceptibility-weighted imaging.

REFERENCES

1. Goldman LW. Principles of CT and CT technology. J Nucl Med Technol 2007;35(3):115–28 [quiz: 129–30].
2. Currie S, Hoggard N, Craven IJ, et al. Understanding MRI: basic MR physics for physicians. Postgrad Med J 2013;89(1050):209–23.
3. Brandao LA, Shiroishi MS, Law M. Brain tumors: a multimodality approach with diffusion-weighted imaging, diffusion tensor imaging, magnetic resonance spectroscopy, dynamic susceptibility contrast and dynamic contrast-enhanced magnetic resonance imaging. Magn Reson Imaging Clin N Am 2013;21(2): 199–239.
4. Cha S. Neuroimaging in neuro-oncology. Neurotherapeutics 2009;6(3):465–77.
5. Law M. Advanced imaging techniques in brain tumors. Cancer Imaging 2009;9(Spec No A):S4–9.
6. Bertholdo D, Watcharakorn A, Castillo M. Brain proton magnetic resonance spectroscopy: introduction and overview. Neuroimaging Clin N Am 2013;23(3): 359–80.
7. Essig M, Nguyen TB, Shiroishi MS, et al. Perfusion MRI: the five most frequently asked clinical questions. AJR Am J Roentgenol 2013;201(3):W495–510.
8. Gerstner ER, Sorensen AG. Diffusion and diffusion tensor imaging in brain cancer. Semin Radiat Oncol 2011;21(2):141–6.
9. Walker C, Baborie A, Crooks D, et al. Biology, genetics and imaging of glial cell tumours. Br J Radiol 2011;84(Spec No 2):S90–106.
10. Park S, Suh YL, Nam DH, et al. Gliomatosis cerebri: clinicopathologic study of 33 cases and comparison of mass forming and diffuse types. Clin Neuropathol 2009;28(2):73–82.
11. Yang S, Wetzel S, Law M, et al. Dynamic contrast-enhanced T2*-weighted MR imaging of gliomatosis cerebri. AJNR Am J Neuroradiol 2002;23(3):350–5.
12. Koeller KK, Rushing EJ. From the archives of the AFIP: oligodendroglioma and its variants: radiologic pathologic correlation. Radiographics 2005;25(6):1669–88.
13. Megyesi JF, Kachur E, Lee DH, et al. Imaging correlates of molecular signatures in oligodendrogliomas. Clin Cancer Res 2004;10(13):4303–6.
14. Spampinato MV, Smith JK, Kwock L, et al. Cerebral blood volume measurements and proton MR spectroscopy in grading of oligodendroglial tumors. AJR Am J Roentgenol 2007;188(1):204–12.
15. Louis DN, Ohgaki H, Wiestler OD, et al. The 2007 WHO classification of tumours of the central nervous system. Acta Neuropathol 2007;114(2):97–109.
16. Tso CL, Freije WA, Day A, et al. Distinct transcription profiles of primary and secondary glioblastoma subgroups. Cancer Res 2006;66(1):159–67.
17. Kannan K, Inagaki A, Silber J, et al. Whole-exome sequencing identifies ATRX mutation as a key molecular determinant in lower-grade glioma. Oncotarget 2012;3(10):1194–203.
18. Combs SE, Rieken S, Wick W, et al. Prognostic significance of IDH-1 and MGMT in patients with glioblastoma: one step forward, and one step back? Radiat Oncol 2011;6:115.
19. Inamasu J, Nakamura Y, Saito R, et al. Rebleeding from a primary brain tumor manifesting as intracerebral hemorrhage (CNN 04/077, revised version). Clin Neurol Neurosurg 2005;108(1):105–8.
20. Weisberg LA. Hemorrhagic primary intracranial neoplasms: clinical-computed tomographic correlations. Comput Radiol 1986;10(2–3):131–6.
21. Osborn AG, Salzman KL, Barkovich AJ. Diagnostic imaging. Brain. 2nd edition. Salt Lake City (UT): Amirsys; 2010.
22. Lee YY, Van Tassel P, Bruner JM, et al. Juvenile pilocytic astrocytomas: CT and MR characteristics. AJR Am J Roentgenol 1989;152(6):1263–70.
23. Strong JA, Hatten HP Jr, Brown MT, et al. Pilocytic astrocytoma: correlation between the initial imaging features and clinical aggressiveness. AJR Am J Roentgenol 1993;161(2):369–72.
24. Rumboldt Z, Camacho DL, Lake D, et al. Apparent diffusion coefficients for differentiation of cerebellar tumors in children. AJNR Am J Neuroradiol 2006; 27(6):1362–9.
25. Pascual-Castroviejo I, Pascual-Pascual SI, Viano J, et al. Posterior fossa tumors in children with neurofibromatosis type 1 (NF1). Childs Nerv Syst 2010; 26(11):1599–603.
26. Jansen MH, Veldhuijzen van Zanten SE, Sanchez Aliaga E, et al. Survival prediction model of children with diffuse intrinsic pontine glioma based on clinical and radiological criteria. Neuro Oncol 2014. [Epub ahead of print].
27. Vallero SG, Bertin D, Basso ME, et al. Diffuse intrinsic pontine glioma in children and adolescents: a single center experience. Childs Nerv Syst 2014; 30(6):1061–6.
28. Lober RM, Cho YJ, Tang Y, et al. Diffusion-weighted MRI derived apparent diffusion coefficient identifies prognostically distinct subgroups of pediatric diffuse intrinsic pontine glioma. J Neurooncol 2014; 117(1):175–82.
29. Conway AE, Reddick WE, Li Y, et al. "Occult" post-contrast signal enhancement in pediatric diffuse intrinsic pontine glioma is the MRI marker of angiogenesis? Neuroradiology 2014;56(5):405–12.
30. Kramm CM, Butenhoff S, Rausche U, et al. Thalamic high-grade gliomas in children: a distinct clinical subset? Neuro Oncol 2011;13(6):680–9.
31. Reardon DA, Gajjar A, Sanford RA, et al. Bithalamic involvement predicts poor outcome among children

with thalamic glial tumors. Pediatr Neurosurg 1998; 29(1):29–35.

32. Perez-Magan E, Campos-Martin Y, Mur P, et al. Genetic alterations associated with progression and recurrence in meningiomas. J Neuropathol Exp Neurol 2012;71(10):882–93.

33. Murovic JA, Chang SD. A literature review of key molecular genetic aberrations in meningiomas: a potential role in the determination of radiosurgery outcomes. World Neurosurg 2014;81(5–6):714–6.

34. Yue Q, Isobe T, Shibata Y, et al. New observations concerning the interpretation of magnetic resonance spectroscopy of meningioma. Eur Radiol 2008; 18(12):2901–11.

35. Zhang H, Rodiger LA, Shen T, et al. Perfusion MR imaging for differentiation of benign and malignant meningiomas. Neuroradiology 2008;50(6):525–30.

36. Blasel S, Jurcoane A, Franz K, et al. Elevated peritumoural rCBV values as a mean to differentiate metastases from high-grade gliomas. Acta Neurochir (Wien) 2010;152(11):1893–9.

37. Crisi G, Orsingher L, Filice S. Lipid and macromolecules quantitation in differentiating glioblastoma from solitary metastasis: a short-echo time single-voxel magnetic resonance spectroscopy study at 3 T. J Comput Assist Tomogr 2013;37(2):265–71.

38. Bradley D, Rees J. Brain tumour mimics and chameleons. Pract Neurol 2013;13(6):359–71.

The Basics of Intraoperative Diagnosis in Neuropathology

 CrossMark

Han S. Lee, MD, PhD*, Tarik Tihan, MD, PhD

KEYWORDS

- Intraoperative diagnosis • Neuropathology • Neurosurgery • Biopsy • Cytologic smear
- Frozen section

ABSTRACT

Intraoperative pathologic consultation continues to be an essential tool during neurosurgical procedures, helping to ensure adequacy of material for achieving a pathologic diagnosis and to guide surgeons. For pathologists, successful consultation with central nervous system lesions involves not only a basic familiarity with the pathologic features of such lesions but also an understanding of their clinical and radiologic context. This review discusses a basic approach to intraoperative diagnosis for practicing pathologists, including preparation for, performance of, and interpretation of an intraoperative neuropathologic evaluation. The cytologic and frozen section features of select examples of common pathologic entities are described.

OVERVIEW

Intraoperative diagnosis has long played an important role in guiding neurosurgical biopsies and resections, and a high degree of accuracy in such rapid diagnoses is the norm.[1] Stereotactic biopsies may yield nondiagnostic tissue in 33% of the first specimens, and intraoperative evaluation of this material helps assure that a sufficient number of biopsies and diagnostic tissue are obtained.[2] Studies suggest that a minimum of 4 core biopsy specimens may be necessary to ensure the highest diagnostic yield ($\geq$89%).[2,3]

Discrepancies between intraoperative diagnoses and final diagnoses may occur in less than 3% of cases.[4] These discrepancies are most commonly encountered with spindle cell lesions, in distinguishing astrocytoma versus oligodendroglioma, in differential diagnosis of lymphoma, grading of tumors, and in distinguishing reactive lesions from neoplasms.[4] Recent advances in neuroradiologic techniques have improved the preoperative understanding of neurosurgical lesions and aid the interpreting pathologist in forming a preoperative differential diagnosis (for a more detailed discussion, see the article by Glastonbury and Tihan elsewhere in this issue). Regardless of the certainty of a radiologic diagnosis, intraoperative evaluation still serves to ensure that the surgically obtained tissue is sufficient enough for accurate diagnosis.

This review discusses an approach to the performance and evaluation of neuropathologic intraoperative diagnoses. First, critical issues in some of the key clinical and radiologic details of the patient and the lesion are presented as well as the necessity for familiarity with the procedure. Some technical insights to intraoperative specimen handling are also provided. Finally, the cytologic and frozen section features of some of the common lesions encountered in general practice are discussed. A more detailed understanding of the clinical, radiologic, and pathologic features of central nervous system (CNS) lesions is referred to other comprehensive sources.[5–7]

Disclosure: The authors have no interests or conflicts to declare.
Neuropathology Division, Department of Anatomic Pathology, University of California, San Francisco, 505 Parnassus Ave, M551, Box 0102, San Francisco, CA 94143, USA
* Corresponding author.
E-mail address: Han.lee@ucsfmedctr.org

surgpath.theclinics.com

PREPARING FOR AN INTRAOPERATIVE DIAGNOSIS: WHAT TO KNOW BEFORE

IS THE PROCEDURE A BIOPSY OR A RESECTION?

The diagnostic goal of intraoperative consultation varies with the type of surgery performed: biopsy or resection. With a biopsy, be it stereotactic core biopsy or open biopsy, intraoperative consultation serves primarily to confirm the presence of diagnostic material in the tissue. A precise diagnosis or grading is typically unnecessary and communicating the presence of "lesional tissue" is often sufficient. However, the potential need for ancillary studies in particular for microbiologic cultures, should be carefully considered. The observation of numerous inflammatory cells should raise the possibility of an infectious/inflammatory process in the differential diagnosis, and communication with the surgeon should include a discussion of tissue submitted for microbiology. Consideration should also be given to whether the pathologic findings are representative of the expected clinical and radiologic abnormalities. In addition, cases often require immunohistochemical work-up, and the presence of quantitatively sufficient tissue is critical when addressing adequacy and communicating this to the surgeon. Acquisition of sufficient amounts of tissue is becoming increasingly important in the current age of molecular pathology, where many molecular/genetic analyses are required as a standard of care rather than a luxury (**Box 1**).

Intraoperative consultation during a neurosurgical procedure not only confirms the presence of lesional tissue but also should serve to help guide a surgeon's approach. Confirmation of the preoperative diagnosis with intraoperative consultation certainly helps support the rationale for the resection of a lesion and informs the surgeon that the management approach has been appropriate.

The intraoperative diagnosis communicated to the surgeon during a definitive procedure typically requires a more specific diagnosis than simply "abnormal tissue." In this context, it is important to distinguish types of lesions for which total resection is not necessarily indicated, as opposed to those that warrant an attempt at gross total resection. The former should prompt strong consideration by the surgeon to limit the extent of resection. Key examples of such lesions include infections, inflammatory lesions such as multiple sclerosis (MS), and some tumors such as malignant lymphoma. Certain neoplastic processes, typically those that respond to radiation therapy and/or chemotherapy, also obviate resection, such as germ cell tumors, Langerhans cell histiocytosis, and small cell carcinoma. In addition, it is also helpful to try to distinguish infiltrating gliomas from gliomas or glioneuronal tumors that are categorized as "circumscribed." Some common examples of such circumscribed primary neoplasms include ganglioglioma, pleomorphic xanthoastrocytoma (PXA), ependymoma, and pilocytic astrocytoma, where gross total resection is usually desirable and achievable. Although gross total resection could be the goal for infiltrating gliomas (and correlates with prognosis), given the diffusely infiltrative nature of these neoplasms and potential involvement of critical structures, gross total resection may not always be practical (**Boxes 2 and 3**).

WHAT ARE THE BASIC CLINICAL AND RADIOLOGIC FEATURES OF THE PATIENT AND LESION?

A basic awareness of the radiologic features of a lesion remains a key part of the understanding of the nature of the disease, and pathologic-radiologic correlation helps confirm whether the tissue evaluated for intraoperative diagnosis is representative. The combination of patient demographics, location of the lesion, and other basic radiologic features form the basis of preoperative diagnosis. Understanding the radioimaging

---

Box 1
Adequacy in a biopsy specimen

1. Pathologically lesional tissue is present.

2. Pathologic features are likely representative of the preoperative differential diagnosis.

3. Adequate amount of tissue is available for ancillary work-up.

Box 2
Typical CNS lesions that do not require gross total resection

Infection and other inflammatory lesions

Demyelination

Lymphoma

Germ cell tumors

Langerhans cell histiocytosis

Small cell carcinoma

Box 3
Common examples of relatively circumscribed glial or glioneuronal neoplasms

Pilocytic astrocytoma

Ganglioglioma/gangliocytoma

Pleomorphic xanthoastrocytoma

Ependymoma/subependymoma

---

features of some of the most common lesions can be helpful to pathologists. The awareness of a patient's clinical history also forms a critical part of constructing a reasonable differential diagnosis. Key elements, such as history of immune deficiency, recent corticosteroid therapy, or any other preoperative treatment, are important examples.

WHAT IS THE LOCATION OF THE LESION?

The location of a lesion should be defined in relation to the compartments of the intracranial space and spinal tissues. The key distinction of intra-axial/intramedullary (present within brain/spinal cord parenchyma) versus extra-axial/extramedullary (arising outside of brain/spinal cord parenchyma) mass defines 2 distinct groups of lesions in the differential diagnosis. Meningiomas and schwannomas typically are extra-axial or extramedullary, whereas gliomas are intra-axial mass lesions. Pathologists should also be aware, however, of the lesions that span both intracranial compartments, wherein the origin is

not clinically clear until the pathology is confirmed. In the spine, the term, *extradural*, describes lesions external to the dura, where soft tissue and bone are the tissues involved. Within the cranial space, distinction of the supratentorial and infratentorial spaces is also critical in constructing a list of possible diagnoses.

A wide variety of primary neoplasms can exist throughout the neuraxis. Certain structures of the neuraxis, however, also impart a specific differential diagnosis that pathologists should recognize. Such sites include the region of the sella turcica (pituitary), the pineal gland, and the intraventricular spaces. Ultimately, a more in-depth understanding of neuropathology allows an understanding of the typical and atypical locations for each CNS lesion (Table 1).

It is impractical for practicing pathologists to have a detailed understanding of neuroradiology. At minimum, pathologists should be aware of the potential significance of certain types of information described in the radiology report. Classic descriptions, such as a "rim-enhancing mass" or "cyst with a solid enhancing nodule," imply particular differential diagnoses that pathologists should consider (Boxes 4 and 5). It is also important to recognize the list of common entities in which such features are observed. Not all rim-enhancing lesions are glioblastomas. The presence of a cyst with a solid mural nodule in the cerebellum classically describes either pilocytic astrocytoma or hemangioblastoma. An understanding of the circumscription of a mass lesion can help define whether or not a neoplasm is diffusely infiltrative. Finally, the presence or

---

Table 1
Subregion-specific differential diagnoses

Typical Mass Lesions of the Sella Turcica and Suprasellar Region	Typical Mass Lesions of the Pineal Gland	Typical Intraventricular Tumors
• Pituitary adenoma • Rathke cleft cyst • Epidermoid/dermoid cyst • Meningioma • Craniopharyngioma • Pituicytoma/spindle cell oncocytoma • Granular cell tumor • Germ cell tumors • Chordoma/chondrosarcoma	• Pineal parenchymal tumors (pineocytoma to pineoblastoma) • Germ cell tumors • Pineal cyst • Papillary tumor of pineal • Gliomas	• Central neurocytoma (lateral ventricle) • Choroid plexus papilloma/carcinoma • Subependymal giant cell astrocytoma • Subependymoma • Ependymoma (4th ventricle) • Meningioma • Parenchymal tumors protruding into ventricle

Basic radiologic features to pay attention to for all lesions
• Circumscription
• Enhancement
• Classic patterns

Box 4
Rim-enhancing lesions

- Glioblastoma
- Metastasis
- Lymphoma (infrequent)
- Abscess
- Multiple Sclerosis (tumefactive)

---

absence of contrast enhancement may have implications for the expected grade of a primary neoplasm. Contrast enhancement is of little value in most low-grade, circumscribed neoplasms because they typically demonstrate enhancement. Some examples are ependymoma, PXA, ganglioglioma, and pilocytic astrocytoma. Among infiltrating gliomas, however, the presence of brisk contrast enhancement implies a higher-grade tumor. When faced with the pathologic features of an infiltrating astrocytoma, the presence of brisk enhancement suggests to pathologists that the lesion is expected to be high grade, and a careful search for mitotic activity, microvascular proliferation, or necrosis is indicated.

TISSUE HANDLING DURING AN INTRAOPERATIVE DIAGNOSIS

In sampling tissue for intraoperative diagnosis, every attempt should be made to save a portion of each specimen for permanent section evaluation, without freezing. Even when additional tissue is undoubtedly expected, there is no guarantee that subsequent tissues will show the same pathologic features. A rough rule of thumb is to try to reserve approximately half of a particular specimen for permanent sections if the initial sample is at least 0.5 cm in the greatest dimension. Furthermore, when faced with a potentially unusual neoplastic process, such as a spindled or small blue cell neoplasm, consideration should also be given for the possibility of an electron microscopic evaluation, and placing some tissue in glutaraldehyde may be indicated.

Box 5
Cystic lesions with enhancing mural nodule

- Pilocytic astrocytoma
- Ganglioglioma
- Pleomorphic xanthoastrocytoma
- Hemangioblastoma

WHEN TO USE CYTOLOGIC SMEAR PREPARATION?

In the intraoperative neuropathologic evaluation, the cytologic smear/squash preparation has long been accepted as a critical component of a complete intraoperative evaluation. The cytologic smear ideally should be performed in every case in conjunction with the standard cryosection (frozen section).[1] The morphologic features provided by each modality complement each other in synthesizing an overall diagnosis. Although the use of cytologic smear preparation alone or frozen section alone may achieve relatively high diagnostic accuracies,[8,9] the combination of the 2 modalities significantly improves the diagnostic rates, resulting in a positive correlation with the final diagnosis in approximately 95% of CNS cases.[10] In cases where tissue is limited, the ability to interpret a cytologic smear preparation as a first step could provide a sufficiently helpful preliminary diagnosis and allow tissue conservation for final diagnosis.

Nuclear and cytoplasmic detail and fibrillary processes are some of the key features that are better viewed on a cytologic smear preparation than a frozen section. The susceptibility of CNS tissue to freezing artifact further underscores the importance of the cytologic smear preparation.

In performing a cytologic smear, only a minimal amount of tissue is necessary, ideally less than 1 mm³. Excessive tissue simply contributes to excessive thickness of the smear and piling of cells. Only moderate pressure should be applied between the glass slides in squashing the tissue. Certain lesions are, by nature, resistant to spreading, and tend to remain in large clumps. Highly gliotic tissues, radiation-treated tissues, and mesenchymal lesions, such as schwannoma, are some common examples in which uniform smears are difficult to achieve. The inability to spread a piece of tissue well during the smear process already provides some degree of information to pathologists. Excess pressure in smearing tissue only serves to crush nuclei and further reduces cytologic detail, thus should be avoided. As with any alcohol-fixed cytologic preparation, immediate immersion of the smear preparation into fixative is essential to minimize air-drying artifacts.

SMALL VERSUS LARGE TISSUE SPECIMENS

Tissues received for intraoperative evaluation range in size from barely 1 to 2 mm to several cubic inches. Both extremes in tissue quantity pose their challenges for pathologists. Stereotactic core biopsies are by their nature small, but the availability of more than one tissue core should afford the opportunity to perform both a cytologic smear as well as a frozen section, while leaving a significant amount of tissue unaltered for permanent section. Situations where the amount of tissue (less than 0.5 cm) is insufficient for cytologic smear preparation, frozen section, and unfrozen permanent section pose a particular challenge for pathologists. Unfortunately, small quantities of tissue are often the norm when a neurosurgeon is working in particularly vulnerable anatomic regions of the CNS, such as the brainstem, spinal cord, or deep gray structures. When faced with such situations, it is a great advantage to be able to perform and intrepret a cytologic smear preparation only, while forgoing or at least postponing a frozen section to preserve tissue. If it becomes impossible to preserve a portion for permanent sections, it is prudent to confirm with the surgeon that the intraoperative diagnosis will potentially change the surgery and that more tissue is forthcoming prior to sampling the entire tissue.

Occasionally, a surgeon provides a particularly large fragment of brain tissue, and the pathologist is faced with the problem of choosing the right area to sample. Understanding the macroscopic features of normal gray and white matter helps to identify the abnormal tissue that should be sampled. When the resection specimen includes both gray and white matter, areas with an indistinct gray-white junction can be sampled to help identify an infiltrative process. Erythematous or hypervascular-appearing tissue (but not blood) is also a good focus for sampling and may harbor higher-grade elements of an infiltrating glioma. When confronted with the possibility of an infiltrating glioma, the white matter should be sampled as infiltrating gliomas show a propensity for spread along white matter tracts.

INTERPRETING THE INTRAOPERATIVE PREPARATION

In this section of the review, the frozen section characteristics and differential diagnosis of some common lesions are discussed. In examining a cytologic smear preparation, 3 general morphologic attributes can be considered:

1. The background of the smear, such as the presence of well-defined glial processes, delicate neuronal processes seen as amorphous eosinophilic material, mesenchymal background, epithelial background, and necrosis
2. The cytology of cells, including nuclear and chromatin features, cytoplasm quality, and association with processes
3. Architectural features that can be seen in smears, including rosettes/pseudorosettes, angiocentric arrangement, or whorls

The fundamental diagnostic algorithm in neuropathology also applies to an intraoperative diagnosis (Fig. 1). The first question should be, "Is the tissue abnormal/lesional?" (eg, "Is it hypercellular?"). If the tissue is abnormal (for instance,

Fig.   1. Intraoperative diagnosis algorithm.

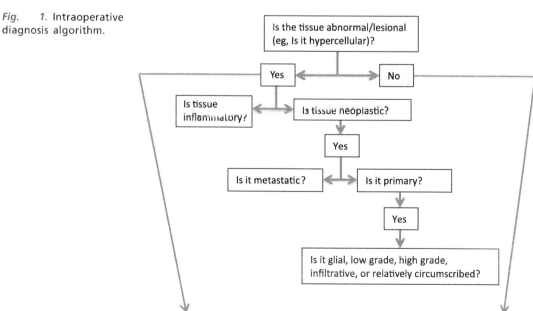

hypercellular), the second question to pose is whether the lesion is neoplastic or inflammatory. If neoplastic, the third inquiry can be whether the tumor is primary or metastasic. Next is the ascertainment of the primary tumor as glial or nonglial. The glial tumors need to be further categorized as low grade, high grade, infiltrative, or circumscribed. Finally, the pathologist should ask, "Is the pathologic diagnosis representative of the clinical and radiologic features?"

NORMAL AND NONDIAGNOSTIC SAMPLES

In determining what is abnormal/lesional, how normal tissue appears must be understood and nonspecific changes recognized.

Samples of CNS tissue, from brain or spinal cord, consist of white matter and/or gray matter, with the cerebral cortex representing a common source of gray matter. Oligodendroglia comprises the predominant cell population in white matter. As such, smears and frozen sections of white matter show a near monomorphic population of cells with uniform small round nuclei (**Fig. 2**A). Although normal CNS tissue appears uniformly thin and well spread on a smear preparation, thickened areas with multiple cell layers may form when abundant tissue is used. Gliotic tissue, with its abundance of glial fibrillary processes, is particularly susceptible to clumping and thickened smears. Such thickened, piled-up tissue may be overinterpreted as hypercellular (see **Fig. 2**B). Care should be taken not to interpret the false hypercellularity and cellular monomorphism seen in such thickened smear preparations of white matter for a neoplasm (eg, oligodendroglioma) or inflammatory infiltrate. Hypercellularity is assessed most easily in a frozen section, when available, and a representative frozen section should confirm the true cellularity of such thickened tissue smears of normal or gliotic brain tissue (see **Fig. 2**C).

Typical smear preparations of gray matter shows a well-spread population of large cells (neurons) intermixed with the small glia (oligodendroglia and astrocytes) and endothelial cells (see **Fig. 2**D). The prominent nucleolus and ample, often triangular-shaped, basophilic cytoplasm forms a readily recognizable morphology for larger neurons (see **Fig. 2**E, F). In smear preparations, the neuronal cytoplasm is often inconspicuous or stripped, and the presence of collections of such large nuclei should not be interpreted as an atypical cell population (see **Fig. 2**E). In smear preparations of any brain or spinal cord tissue, a well-formed background of cotton candy–like amorphous eosinophilic material is apparent, representing the delicate meshwork of the neuronal

processes of CNS parenchyma (see **Fig. 2**A, B, D, E). Well-defined fine lines also may be seen and represent glial fibrillary processes.

When confronted with a sample from the posterior fossa, pathologists should remember the possibility of sampling of cerebellar cortex, with its densely cellular small round blue cell appearance imparted by the internal granule cell layer (**Fig. 3**A). Particularly in smears, as well as in minute frozen section samples, a small round blue cell neoplasm, such as medulloblastoma, may be considered when viewing such material. The nuclear uniformity, absence of cell proliferation or cell death, and presence of occasional large neurons representing Purkinje cells are clues to the true identity of the tissue (see **Fig. 3**B). A frozen section of ample size generally confirms the source of tissue as well (see **Fig. 3**C).

Nonspecific histopathologic changes that may be seen in a sample include necrosis, astrogliosis, and perivascular chronic inflammation (see **Fig. 3**D). Although these types of changes usually are part of a particular pathologic process, in the absence of additional, more specific evidence, such morphology should be considered nondiagnostic and surgeons should be prompted for additional material.

INFILTRATING GLIOMAS AND OTHER COMMON GLIAL NEOPLASMS

Infiltrating gliomas comprise the most common category of primary neoplasms arising in the CNS, and include

1. Diffuse astrocytoma (World Health Organization [WHO] grade II)[5]
2. Anaplastic astrocytoma (grade III)
3. Glioblastoma (grade IV)
4. Oligodendroglioma (grade II)
5. Anaplastic oligodendroglioma (grade III)

At the lower end of tumor cellularity, as may be seen at the periphery of any of these diffusely infiltrative neoplasms, diagnosis often represents a significant challenge. By the infiltrative nature of these neoplasms, particularly of grade II astrocytoma, the predominant cellular component in a particular tissue sample is often non-neoplastic, and identifying the handful of neoplastic astrocytes intermixed within poses a difficult diagnostic challenge (**Fig. 4**A).

Infiltrating Astrocytoma

Diagnosable, infiltrating astrocytoma is recognized as an increased population of atypical cells, with elongate to irregular naked nuclei and coarse

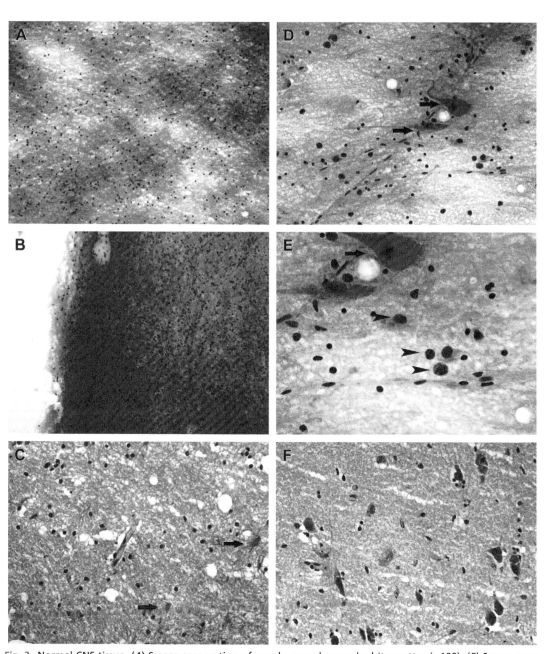

Fig. 2. Normal CNS tissue. (*A*) Smear preparation of evenly spread normal white matter (×100). (*B*) Smear preparation of white matter in a thickened area showing false increase in cellularity (×100). (*C*) Frozen section of white matter, with a few reactive astrocytes (*arrows*) (×200). (*D*) Smear preparation of evenly spread normal gray matter, with intact large neurons (*arrows*) and amorphous eosinophilic/pink background of fine neuronal processes (×200). (*E*) Smear preparation of gray matter with intact large neurons (*arrow*) and stripped neuronal nuclei (*arrowheads*) (×400). (*F*) Frozen section of cortical gray matter with neurons and scattered glia (×200).

chromatin, in a background of CNS tissue (see Fig. 4B). A haphazard arrangement of tumor cells is present, without definable architectural features. When tumor represents an overall minority of the cells in the tissue, the presence of clusters of such atypical cells with naked nuclei aids in their recognition (see Fig. 4D). As with most gliomas, glial fibrillary process are generally well represented and best seen on smear preparations (see Fig. 4C) although, in poorly differentiated examples of glioblastoma, they are often sparse or lacking. The cytologic background generally includes not only glial fibrillary processes (see Fig. 4C, upper right corner) but also the

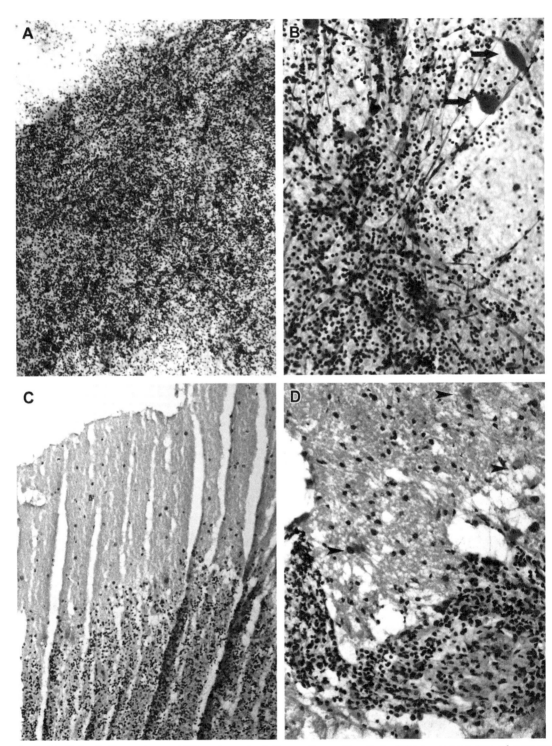

Fig. 3. (*A–C*) Cerebellar cortex and (*D*) perivascular inflammation with gliosis. (*A*) Low-power view of a smear preparation of cerebellar cortex, with abundant internal granule cells mimicking a small blue cell proliferation (×100). (*B*) Moderate-power view of cerebellar cortex smear, showing uniform small round nuclei and several large Purkinje neurons (*arrows*). (*C*) Frozen section confirms normal architecture of cerebellar cortex, with hypocellular molecular layer, densely cellular internal granule cell layer and Purkinje cells at the interface (×100). (*D*) Frozen section of a focus of perivascular lymphocytic infiltrate and adjacent astrogliosis, a nonspecific pattern (reactive astrocytes [*arrowheads*]) (×200).

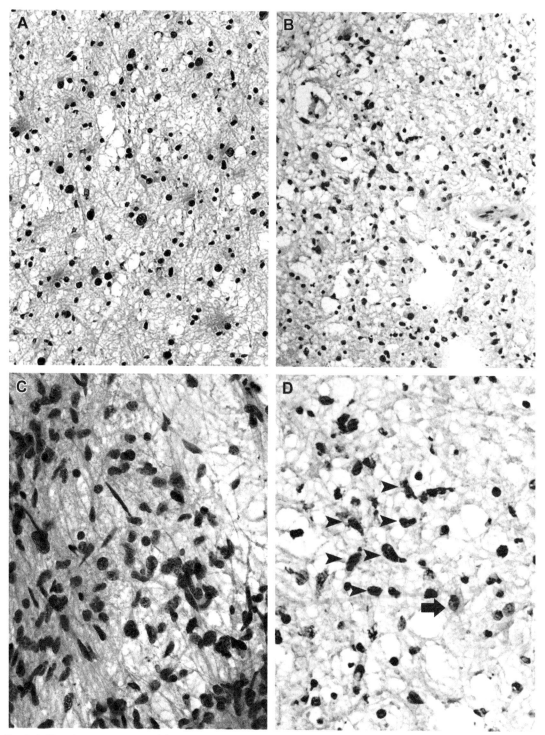

Fig. 4. Infiltrating astrocytoma. (*A*) Frozen section showing mildly increased cellularity of gray matter in a subtle case of astrocytoma (×200). (*B*) Frozen section of an area of infiltrating astrocytoma with more evident tumor hypercellularity. Brain parenchyma is still evident in the background (×200). (*C*) High-power view of a smear of an infiltrating astrocytoma, with a predominance of atypical astrocytic nuclei, associated with glial fibrillary processes (*upper right corner*). Eosinophilic material suggesting CNS tissue is intermixed (*lower left corner*) (×400). (*D*) High-power frozen section view demonstrating a cluster of atypical astrocytic naked nuclei (*arrowheads*) that is diagnostic of tumor. Background CNS tissue is evident and includes neurons (*arrow*) (×400).

amorphous eosinophilic material of CNS parenchyma (see Fig. 4C, lower left corner), a feature further suggesting an infiltrative morphologic pattern. The presence of glial fibrillary processes alone does not denote a glioma, however, because astrogliosis itself also produces such a pattern. In addition, occasionally, a nonglial neoplasm inciting a gliotic reaction presents a cytologic picture of a neoplastic proliferation admixed with glial fibrillary processes. Such a picture may be seen particularly with CNS lymphoma, in occasions where they show extensive infiltrative growth.

Once the histologic pattern of an infiltrating astrocytoma is recognized, a search for high-grade features should be performed. Multiple mitoses in an infiltrating astrocytoma denote WHO grade III whereas necrosis or microvascular proliferation is diagnostic of grade IV (WHO reference). Given the presence of such lesional tissue with evidence of an astrocytic neoplasm, it can then be asked whether the diagnosis and grade considered are representative of the clinical and radiologic features. Infiltrating astrocytomas can occur throughout the CNS and in all age ranges, but increased age should raise a suspicion for the possibility of a high-grade tumor. An ill-defined T2 fluid-attenuated inversion recovery (FLAIR) hyperintense mass lesion by MRI fits the picture of an infiltrating glioma, and the presence of contrast enhancement should denote high grade (at least WHO grade III) as well. A minority subset of nonenhancing infiltrating gliomas are high grade.

Circumscribed Glial or Glioneuronal Neoplasms

Additionally, particularly in younger patients (pediatric or young adults), the alternative possibility that the neoplastic astrocytes are part of a circumscribed low-grade glial or glioneuronal neoplasm should also be considered. Such examples include pilocytic astrocytoma, ganglioglioma and PXA. In small specimens, areas of these circumscribed neoplasms can be indistinguishable from an infiltrating astrocytoma, because some degree of microscopic infiltration is often present in them as well.

Further clues to these possibilities include radiologic features indicating a circumscribed, cystic, and solid-enhancing lesion based in the hemispheric cortices (PXA and ganglioglioma) or in the cerebellum and spinal cord (pilocytic). Histologic clues that the lesion may not be an infiltrating glioma include the presence of eosinophilic granular bodies (Fig. 5A, B), frequently seen in both ganglioglioma and PXA, as well as Rosenthal fibers within the tumor (see Fig. 5C, E), often seen in pilocytic astrocytomas. In gangliogliomas, noting the presence of large, atypical cells somewhat resembling neurons, in addition to the (usually) astrocytic population, further suggests the diagnosis (see Fig. 5A, B). Cytologic smears of pilocytic astrocytoma are typified by uniform neoplastic nuclei accompanied by a background consisting predominantly of dense collections of long strait hairlike fibrillary processes (see Fig. 5D). A background of brain parenchyma may be inapparent. With the exception of the anaplastic variants of PXA and ganglioglioma, mitotic activity should be inconspicuous to rare in these neoplasms. In addition, as may be seen in cystic CNS lesions, microvascular proliferation may be present in these neoplasms, is a feature seen in the cyst wall, and does not denote a high-grade neoplasm.

Rosenthal fibers are not pathognomic for a neoplasm (such as pilocytic astrocytoma) because they are also seen in some chronically gliotic/reactive tissues. Such piloid gliosis is a common feature in the spinal cord and hypothalamus, particularly as a reaction to vascular lesions and craniopharyngiomas. Distinguishing piloid gliosis from pilocytic astrocytoma in small specimens often poses a challenge (Box 6).

These alternative possibilities when considering an astrocytic neoplasm are an example of the importance of correlation with the clinical and radiologic features.

Diagnostic Terminology

Diagnostic terminology that may be considered at the time of frozen section include "infiltrating astrocytoma, no high-grade features," "astrocytic neoplasm," "glioma," or "low-grade glial or glioneuronal tumor," depending on the degree of certainty as to the classification and grade. Given the problems of sample bias in a small specimen, it is not always possible to distinguish an infiltrating astrocytoma from the low-grade circumscribed neoplasms, particularly at the time of intraoperative diagnosis. It is fully reasonable for a pathologist to suggest a differential diagnosis in such situations.

Box 6
Lesions commonly associated with piloid gliosis

- Hemangioblastoma

- Cavernous angioma

- Arteriovenous malformation

- Craniopharyngioma

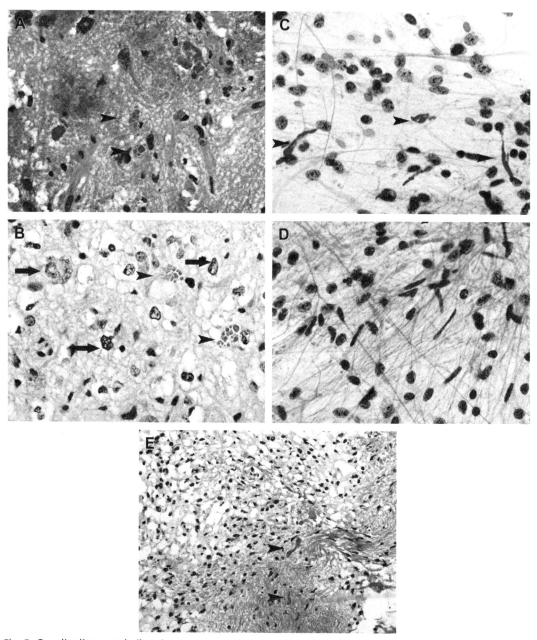

Fig. 5. Ganglioglioma and pilocytic astrocytoma. Frozen section (*A*) and permanent section (*B*) of ganglioglioma with visible eosinophilic granular bodies (*arrowheads*) and atypical ganglion cells (*arrows*) (×400). (*C*) Cytologic smear of a pilocytic astrocytoma demonstrating Rosenthal fibers (*arrowheads*) (×400). (*D*) Cytologic smear of a pilocytic astrocytoma showing the predominant background of hairlike fibrillary processes. (*E*) Frozen section shows Rosenthal fibers (*arrowheads*) associated with a glial tumor with loosely textured area of tumor (*upper left*) adjacent to a compact area (*lower right*) (×200).

Ultimately, immunohistochemical evaluation may be necessary to help with more specific classification. In this regard, immunohistochemistry for mutant IDH1(R132H) has become particularly helpful in confirming classification as an infiltrating glioma.

Ependymomas

Not only are fibrillary processes associated with a neoplasm a feature seen in astrocytic neoplasms but such processes are also usually present in ependymomas (**Fig. 6**B). The distinctive perivascular pseudorosettes are most apparent in frozen

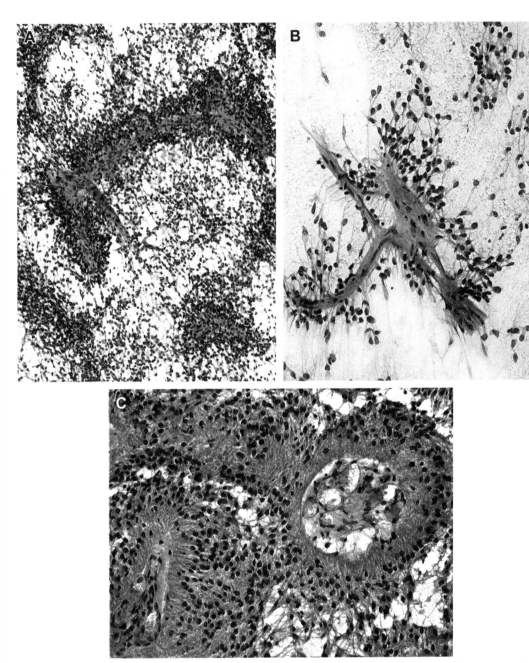

Fig. 6. Ependymoma. (*A*) Low-power view of a smear preparation, demonstrating tumor cells arranged along, but not within, blood vessels (×100). (*B*) At moderate power, glial fibrillary processes are visible, often extending to the vessel walls. Tumor nuclei are uniform, ovoid with fine chromatin (×200). (*C*) Frozen section well illustrates the consistent perivascular pseudorosettes (×200).

section (see **Fig. 6**C) and are often also discernible on the cytologic smear (see **Fig. 6**A), where tumor cells seem to collect in a zone around vessels, while respecting the boundaries of the vessels themselves, unlike in lymphoma. Ependymal tumor cells uniformly show oval nuclei with fine, speckled chromatin. Ependymomas are sharply circumscribed masses, and, unlike PXA, ganglioglioma, and pilocytic astrocytoma, microscopic areas of infiltration are generally entirely absent. Given the presence of these cytologic features and well-developed architecture of perivascular pseudorosettes, a specific diagnosis can usually be rendered intraoperatively, including with small specimens. A well defined, homogeneously enhancing mass associated with the 4th ventricle or within the spinal cord is the typical radiologic picture for WHO grade II cellular ependymomas.

Oligodendroglioma

Oligodendroglioma represents another form of infiltrating glioma, characterized by a relatively uniform population of round nuclei with fine chromatin

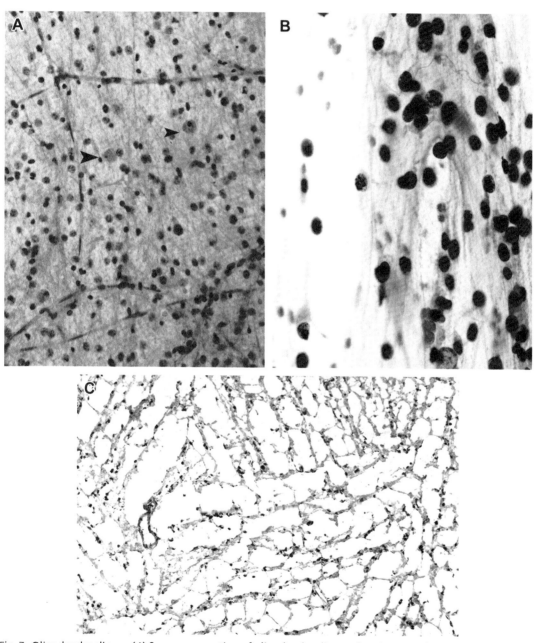

Fig. 7. Oligodendroglioma. (*A*) Smear preparation of oligodendroglioma, showing a predominant population of cells with uniform round nuclei that are larger than typical non-neoplastic oligodendroglia. Chromatin shows less coarseness and hyperchromasia than astrocytic neoplasms. Branching delicate chicken-wire vasculature is often evident on the smear preparations as well. Background brain tissue is evident, including scattered preexisting neurons (*arrowheads*) (×200). (*B*) A richly myxoid example of oligodendroglioma is demonstrated by smear preparation (×400). (*C*) A similar myxoid example is shown by frozen section, with extensive freezing artifact typical of myxoid tissues (×100). Other tumors resembling oligodendroglioma should be considered when faced with such a round-cell predominant pattern, including DNET.

and often accompanied by an arborizing network of fine vessels. Neoplastic oligodendroglia are typically larger than the resident non-neoplastic oligodendroglia that populate white matter, a futher cytologic clue that contributes to the diagnosis. These features are well demonstrated on smear preparations (Fig. 7A). The characteristic fried egg histologic appearance is usually not demonstrated on frozen section or smear preparation, given it is the product of histologic artifact. Being an infiltrative neoplasm, CNS tissue, including occasional neurons, is often visible in the background (see Fig. 7A). Given its morphologic presentation as a proliferation of uniform round nuclei, it is particularly important to exclude the possibility that these cells may be mononuclear inflammatory cells or, in particular, macrophages. Reactive, mature lymphocyes are generally distinguishable by their smaller and denser nuclei. Identification of ample, well-defined, and pale cytoplasm helps identify a macrophage population, a feature better seen on cytologic preparations than frozen sections.

At times, oligodendrogliomas, as well as several other glial and glioneuronal neoplasms, show variable amounts of myxoid tissue (see Fig. 7B), a feature that exacerbates the problem of freezing artifact (see Fig. 7C). Such freezing artifact, with its exaggerated empty spaces, results in an underestimation of the degree of cellularity of the tissue. The identification of myxoid tissue in a tissue sample should be a strong clue for the presence of a primary CNS neoplasm, because it is virtually never seen in reactive processes of the CNS.

Oligodendroglioma has a strong predilection for the cerebral hemispheres (supratentorial brain), and the diagnosis should be doubted when the lesion originates in the posterior fossa, spinal cord, or ventricles. Several other neoplasms may morphologically mimic oligodendroglioma, including central neurocytoma (lateral ventricles), clear cell ependymoma, dysembroplastic neuroepithelial tumor (DNET), and some pilocytic astrocytomas (Box 7). In addition, the distinction between infiltrating astrocytoma and oligodendroglioma is not always apparent, given the often subjective morphologic interpretation of nuclear shape and hyperchromasia.

Glioblastoma Versus Metastasis Versus Lymphoma

In the context of infiltrating gliomas (and not other types of gliomas), the presence of contrast enhancement by MRI correlates with higher grade: WHO grade III or IV.

> **Box 7**
> **Lesions resembling oligodendroglioma**
>
> - Central neurocytoma (lateral ventricles, noninfiltrative)
> - Clear cell ependymoma (noninfiltrative)
> - DNET
> - Pilocytic astrocytoma (Rosenthal fibers, intratentorial)
> - Infiltrating astrocytoma
> - Macrophage-rich lesions

Rim enhancement in particular, with its constituent central necrosis, typically denotes a glioblastoma. Other high-grade neoplasms, however, including metastasis and lymphoma, may present similarly. This trio represents a basic and important differential diagnosis of high-grade neoplasms involving the CNS. In addition, non-neoplastic lesions, such as abscess and tumefactive multiple sclerosis lesions, can show similar radiologic features (Box 4).

The overall cellularity and nuclear atypia seen in areas of glioblastoma can vary considerably. When densely cellular, thick clumpy smear preparations may result (Fig. 8A). In such areas, it may be difficult to discern the type of neoplastic cells involved (see Fig. 8B). Identifying less dense areas (see Fig. 8D) and viewing the periphery of the large tissue clumps (see Fig. 8C) help identify the typical astrocytic morphology of hyperchromatic elongate nuclei and also help discern the well-defined glial processes and background eosinophilic parenchymal tissue. The presence of tumor necrosis and/or microvascular proliferation enables grading of an infiltrating astrocytoma as a WHO grade IV tumor (glioblastoma). Microvascular proliferation can often be identified on a smear preparation as a bulbous collection of many overlapping and haphazardly oriented nuclei, attached to a recognizable vessel (see Fig. 8E). Care should be taken that the many smooth muscle nuclei of an arteriole or a small artery are not interpreted as microvascular proliferation. Frozen sections facilitate recognition of microvascular proliferation (see Fig. 8F). Initial operative specimens may sample the less cellular periphery of a glioblastoma, where the features may at best suggest a lower-grade astrocytoma of low cellularity. Given the context of a rim-enhancing lesion and implication for a high-grade neoplasm, a pragmatic and facile approach is to consider such subtle specimens as simply nondiagnostic, for the purposes of intraoperative diagnosis.

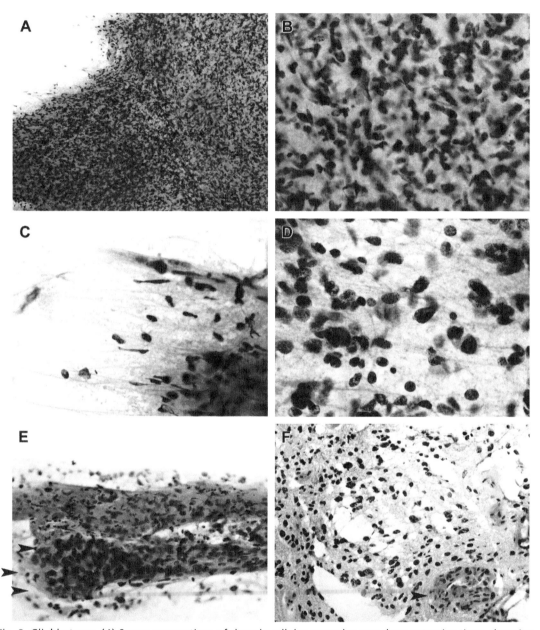

Fig. 8. Glioblastoma. (*A*) Smear preparations of densely cellular examples may show extensive tissue clumping (×100). (*B*) The type of neoplastic process may be difficult to discern when examining the center of thick clumps (×400). (*C*) Viewing the periphery of large tissue clumps can better discern the morphology of tumor cells and the presence of glial processes as part of tumor (×400). (*D*) Thinly spread areas of the smear also allow recognition of the astrocytic morphology of tumor cells, with hyperchromatic and elongate to irregular nuclei. The presence of well-defined fibrillary processes in these areas is also consistent with an astrocytoma (×400). (*E*) Microvascular proliferation may be identified in a cytologic smear as a bulbous projection consisting of haphazardly arranged crowded nuclei (×200). (*F*) Microvascular proliferation on a tissue section is seen as a sharply circumscribed tight collection of overlapping nuclei, with the vessel lumen often obscured (×200).

By far, carcinomas form the most common type of metastatic neoplasm, with melanoma following in frequency. With rare exception, metastases are characterized by a highly compact growth pattern and a sharply defined brain interface.

Typical cytopathologic features of carcinoma help identify them in the brain as well, with cohesive clusters of cells containing variable amounts of cytoplasm. In both smear preparations and frozen section, the lack of infiltrative growth is

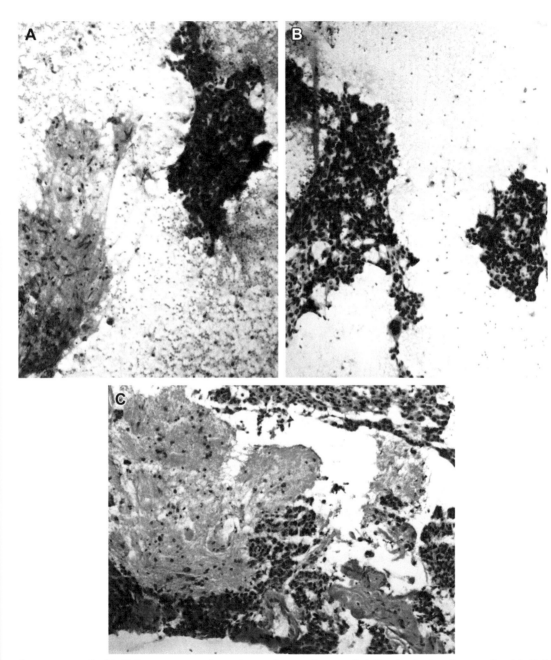

Fig. 9. Metastasis. (*A, B*) Smear preparations of a carcinoma show well-defined cohesive clusters of epithelioid cells that is separate from the CNS tissue that may be present (*left side* [*A*]) (×100). (*C*) Frozen section illustrates the sharply defined interface of tumor and CNS tissue, often containing gliotic tissue (×100).

readily apparent. In smear preparations, tight clusters of tumor cells are seen as distinct from the CNS tissue that may be present (Fig. 9A, B). Glial fibrillary processes are absent in areas of tumor, although the adjacent areas for brain are often gliotic. Frozen sections that include interface with adjacent brain demonstrate the sharp demarcation (see Fig. 9C). Depending on the type of carcinoma, morphologic features, such as gland

formation or squamous differentiation, also facilitate diagnosis. Although cohesive growth is often not a feature of melanoma, the sharp distinction with adjacent brain helps suggest its metastatic nature in the CNS.

The intraoperative diagnosis of lymphoma may have a critical bearing on a surgery, because the diagnosis precludes the need for complete resection. The vast majority of primary CNS lymphomas are diffuse large B-cell type.[5] Cytologic smear preparations often show sufficient features for a specific intraoperative diagnosis and are usually superior to frozen sections. A well-spread dyshesive population of atypical round nuclei is present, often without associated brain tissue intermingling among tumor cells (**Fig. 10**A). At high-power magnification, the tumor nuclei show cytomorphologic features of large B cells, with vesicular, open chromatin; distinct nucleoli;

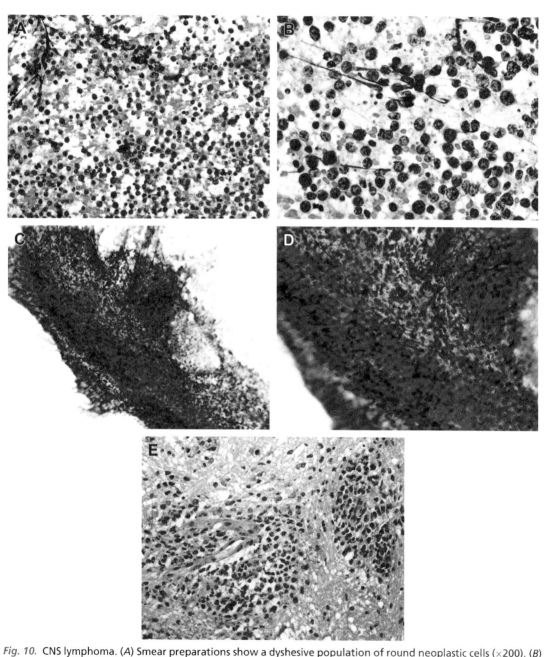

Fig. 10. CNS lymphoma. (*A*) Smear preparations show a dyshesive population of round neoplastic cells (×200). (*B*) At high power, cytologic features typical of large B cells become apparent. Streaks of smeared nuclear material, increased proliferative activity, karyorhectic nuclei, and lymphoglandular bodies are usually present, and an eosinophilic background suggesting CNS parenchyma is often absent (×400). (*C*) Smear preparations readily demonstrate the typical angiocentricity of CNS lymphoma, with long vessels encompassed by tumor cells (×100). (*D*) Close examination of these vessels show tumor cells occupying the walls of blood vessels (×200). (*E*) Angiocentric growth may be seen in frozen sections (×200), but in some cases, a nonspecific appearance of formless sheets of a poorly differentiated neoplasm may predominate.

and on occasion recognizable cytoplasm (see **Fig. 10B**). The background often includes lympho-glandular bodies (see **Fig. 10B**) and, occasionally, tingible body macrophages are also present. The distinctive angiocentric growth pattern of CNS lymphoma is best seen on a smear preparation.

The low-power appearance of tumor cells collecting along tubular structures suggests angiocentric growth (see **Fig. 10C**). High-power view of these vessels should reveal the close relationship of lymphoma cells with the vessels. Tumor cells present within the walls of blood vessels, and not simply

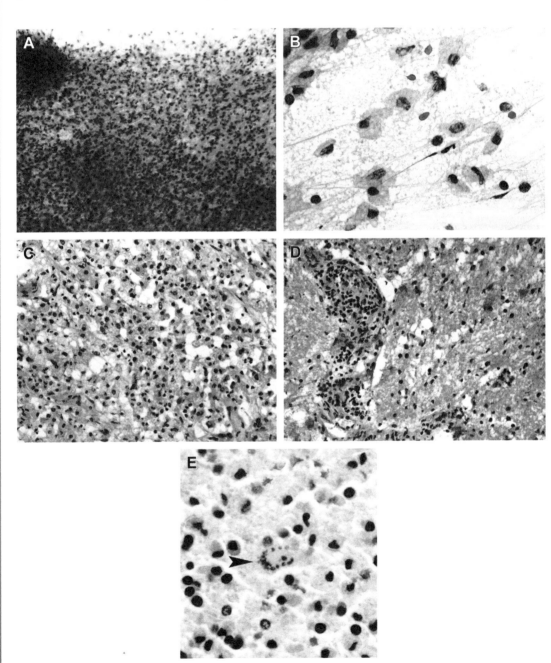

Fig. 11. Macrophage infiltrate of MS. (*A*) Low-power view of cytologic smear shows large clumps of cells suggesting a hypercellular lesion of uncertain classification (×100). (*B*) High-power view away from clumped areas reveal macrophages (×400). (*C*) Frozen section confirms a hypercellular lesion, but its identification as a macrophage infiltrate can be difficult to be certain (×200). (*D*) Adjacent areas show perivascular lymphocytic inflammation and astrogliosis (×200). (*E*) Creutzfeld cells (*arrowhead*), consisting of astrocytes with fragmented nuclei, are a common but nonspecific feature in inflammatory lesions (×400).

around the vessels, is a characteristic feature of the angiocentric growth pattern of CNS lymphoma (see **Fig. 10D**). Frozen sections often show a poorly differentiated malignancy, in which the angiocentric growth pattern may or may not be apparent (see **Fig. 10E**). Although a solid growth pattern is seen in most cases, extensively infiltrative growth can also be seen with CNS lymphomas, with neoplastic lymphocytes intermixed within CNS parenchyma. Given the presence of these morphologic features in a sample, the intraoperative diagnosis of lymphoma is achievable. When lymphoma becomes a clinical or pathologic consideration, pathologists should be aware of any recent corticosteroid therapy, because corticosteroid therapy results in rapid destruction of the lymphocytic population. What remains may be a nonspecific pattern of few lymphocytes, macrophages, and necrosis. Identifying an atypical lymphoid population in this context is often a fruitless task.

Multiple Sclerosis and Macrophage-Rich Lesions

Although the vast majority of MS cases are diagnosed clinically, a subset of those presenting with a single, tumefactive, mass lesion may require pathologic confirmation. In these cases, the clinical and radiologic features do not readily distinguish a neoplasm from a lesion of MS. The typical morphologic features of an active MS plaque can be described as a macrophage-rich lesion, with a cellular infiltrate consisting predominantly of macrophages. A macrophage-rich histologic pattern can be seen in a variety of lesions, however, ranging from infectious to inflammatory to neoplastic (treated lymphoma). In the case of MS, the pathologic pattern includes a perivascular lymphocytic infiltrate and astrogliosis (**Fig. 11D**). Sharply defined zones of demyelination can be identified on permanent section evaluation with Luxol fast blue stain and an axonal stain. Creutzfeldt cells (see **Fig. 11E**), consisting of fragmented astrocytic nuclei, are a feature that is classically described in inflammatory lesions, such as MS, but are not specific.

Both cytologic smear and frozen section preparations of macrophage-rich lesions present as a dense infiltrate of cells with round nuclei and ample cytoplasm (see **Fig. 11A, C**). The identity of this infiltrate as consisting of macrophages may not be readily apparent, particularly on frozen section. Given the similar morphology, mistaking a macrophage population for an oligodendroglial proliferation is readily done when viewing the poor morphology of a frozen section. Examination of

the periphery of tissue clumps and of a dispersed population of cells in a smear preparation should, however, show the recognizable morphology of macrophages (see **Fig. 11B**). When faced with a macrophage infiltrate, pathologists should seek to ensure that the infiltrate is not simply a reaction to an area of tumor necrosis. In addition, given the presence of perivascular lymphocytes, a careful evaluation for an atypical lymphocyte subpopulation is also in order. Although macrophage-rich lesions do not represent a specific pattern, given the persistence of this morphology in the tissue sample, this can be considered lesional tissue for the purposes of biopsy adequacy, albeit lesional tissue that requires further evaluation on permanent section to attempt to identify the etiology. Full pathologic evaluation of these lesions typically entails excluding an infectious process, demyelination, and lymphoma. In the absence of more specific features, an intraoperative diagnosis of "macrophage-rich lesion" is appropriate. Consideration may be given for microbiologic cultures (**Box 8**).

Pituitary Adenoma

A variety of mass lesions are peculiar to the sella turcica (pituitary fossa) and suprasellar region. Resections for suspected pituitary adenomas are a common neurosurgical procedure and the most common indication for surgery in this region. Pituitary adenomas are histologically recognized by the accompanying loss of the normal lobular/acinar architecture (**Fig. 12C**) of the anterior pituitary gland, combined usually with a monomorphic appearance of its pituitary cells. The tumor architecture is variable but includes formless sheets as well as trabecular growth (see **Fig. 12D**). The characteristic cytologic features is of a predominantly dispersed, dyshesive population of monomorphic cells showing the typical bland neuroendocrine nuclear features (see **Fig. 12B**).

Box 8
Macrophage-rich lesions in CNS

- MS and other demyelinative lesions
- Progressive multifocal leukoencephalopathy
- Treated lymphoma
- Infarct
- Fungal infection
- Atypical bacterial infection
- Toxoplasmosis
- Histiocytosis

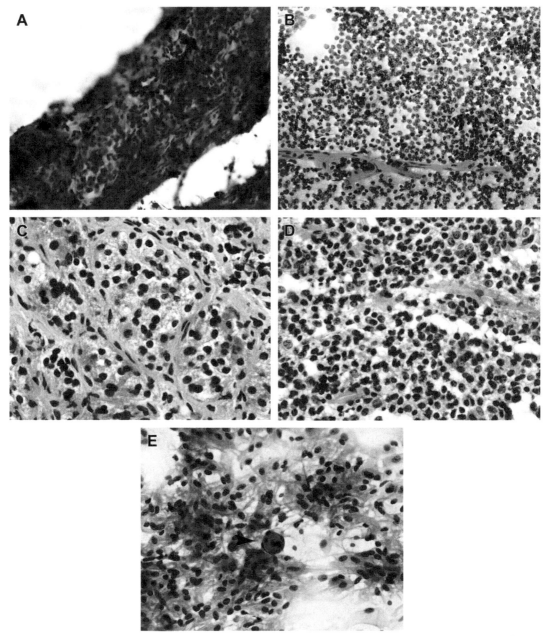

Fig. 12. Pituitary adenoma. (A) Smears of non-neoplastic anterior pituitary tissue show large clumps of tissue from which few anterior pituitary cells are extracted (×100). (B) In contrast, smears of pituitary adenoma show a predominantly dispersed pattern of spread on the slide, consisting of a monomorphic population of pituitary cells (×100). (C) Frozen sections of non-neoplastic pituitary also demonstrate the intact architecture of lobules lined by delicate fibrovascular tissue and frequently heterogeneous appearance of cells in non-neoplastic anterior pituitary (×400). (D) The lack of lobular architecture and monomorphism is readily seen in frozen sections of pituitary adenomas (×400). (E) Meningiomas extending into the pituitary region may be mistaken for pituitary adenoma, given the common epithelioid features. Recognizable features of meningioma, such as whorls (arrowhead), psammoma bodies, and nuclear pseudoinclusions, help to identify this lesion. Smear preparations of meningioma generally show clustered cell groups rather than a dispersed pattern (×400).

This contrasts with the lack of spread of non-neoplastic anterior pituitary cells that are trapped in the fine fibrovascular meshwork of the anterior pituitary (see **Fig. 12**A). The presence of these cytologic features alone is sufficient for the diagnosis of pituitary adenoma. Occasionally, meningiomas of the skull base may involve the sella turcica and form an important morphologic differential diagnosis of an epithelioid neoplasm in this region. When present, meningothelial features, such as whorls (see **Fig. 12**E), psammoma bodies, and syncytial groups of cells, readily distinguish meningioma from pituitary adenomas. Typical cytologic features include spread of the tumor into small clusters and large clumps of cells with broad cytoplasm (see **Fig. 12**E), contrasting with the dispersed population of cells with minimal cytoplasm that describes most adenomas. The broadly spread cytoplasm of individual meningothelial cells also contrasts with the typical indistinct cytoplasm in adenomas.

REFERENCES

1. Folkerth RD. Smears and frozen sections in the intraoperative diagnosis of central nervous system lesions. Neurosurg Clin N Am 1994;5:1–18.

2. Brainard JA, Prayson RA, Barnett GH. Frozen section evaluation of stereotactic brain biopsies: diagnostic yield at the stereotactic target position in 188 cases. Arch Pathol Lab Med 1997;121:481.

3. Jain D, Sharma MC, Sarkar C, et al. Correlation of diagnostic yield of stereotactic brain biopsy with number of bits and site of the lesion. Brain Tumor Pathol 2006;23:71–5.

4. Plesec TP, Prayson RA. Frozen section discrepancy in the evaluation of central nervous system tumors. Arch Pathol Lab Med 2007;131:1532–40.

5. Louis DN, Ohgaki H, Wiestler OD, et al, editors. WHO classification of tumors of the central nervous system. Lyon (France): IARC Press; 2007.

6. Perry A, Brat D. Practical surgical neuropathology. A diagnostic approach. Philadelphia: Churchill Livingstone Elsevier; 2010.

7. Burger PC, Scheithauer BW. Tumors of the central nervous system. AFIP atlas of tumor pathology. Fourth series. Washington, DC: American Registry of Pathology, ARP Press; 2007.

8. Roessler K, Dietrich W, Kitz K. High diagnostic accuracy of cytologic smears of central nervous system tumors. A 15 year experience based on 4172 patients. Acta Cytol 2002;46:667–74.

9. Firlik KS, Martinez AJ, Lunsford LD. Use of cytological preparations for the intraoperative diagnosis of stereotactically obtained brain biopsies: a 19-year experience and survey of neuropathologists. J Neurosurg 1999;91:454–8.

10. Martinez AJ, Pollack I, Hall WA, et al. Touch preparations in the rapid intraoperative diagnosis of central nervous system lesions. A comparison with frozen sections and paraffin-embedded sections. Mod Pathol 1998;1:378–84.

Practical Molecular Pathologic Diagnosis of Infiltrating Gliomas

CrossMark

Melike Pekmezci, MD[a], Arie Perry, MD[a,b],*

KEYWORDS

- Glioma • Infiltrating glioma • Genetic • Epigenetic • Molecular • Isocitrate dehydrogenase
- Epidermal growth factor receptor • Alternative lengthening of telomeres

ABSTRACT

Recent advances in molecular diagnostics have led to better understanding of glioma tumorigenesis and biology. Numerous glioma biomarkers with diagnostic, prognostic, and predictive value have been identified. Although some of these markers are already part of the routine clinical management of glioma patients, data regarding others are limited and difficult to apply routinely. In addition, multiple methods for molecular subclassification have been proposed either together with or as an alternative to the current morphologic classification and grading scheme. This article reviews the literature regarding glioma biomarkers and offers a few practical suggestions.

OVERVIEW

Gliomas account for 20% of all primary central nervous system (CNS) neoplasms and 80% of all malignant CNS tumors.[1] They are typically assigned a histologic subtype and grade according to the most recent World Health Organization (WHO) International Classification of Diseases scheme, based purely on morphologic features.[2] Infiltrating gliomas are classified as astrocytic, oligodendroglial, and mixed and are graded from II through IV. Glioblastoma (astrocytoma, WHO grade IV), the most common primary CNS malignancy in adults, continues to be one of the most lethal tumors, with 1-year and 2-year survival rates of 35% and 14%, respectively.[1] CNS neoplasms are the most common solid tumor of childhood, and the broad category of glioma accounts for 53% of CNS tumors in children ages 0 to 14 years and 37% in adolescents ages 15 to 19. For children ages 0 to 14 years, pilocytic astrocytomas, embryonal tumors, and malignant glioma, not otherwise specified, account for 18%, 15%, and 14%, respectively.

Recent advances in molecular pathology have provided additional diagnostic, prognostic, and predictive biomarkers, leading to alternative classification methods beyond morphology. Additionally, genomic and epigenetic studies have shown that even relatively homogeneous histologic groups (eg, glioblastoma) may be divided into multiple distinct molecular subsets, whereas a single molecular aberration may be seen in more than one histologic tumor type. This review summarizes common alterations that are variably used in the diagnosis of infiltrating gliomas.

1P AND 19Q CODELETION

Concomitant loss of chromosomes 1p and 19q due to an unbalanced centromeric translocation t(1;19)(q10;p10) is one of the best studied molecular alterations in gliomas and is strongly associated with oligodendroglial morphology and improved

This project did not receive funding support.

The authors do not have any conflict of interest.

[a] Division of Neuropathology, Department of Pathology, University of California, San Francisco, 505 Parnassus Avenue, #M551, Box 0102, San Francisco, CA 94143, USA; [b] Department of Neurological Surgery, University of California, San Francisco, 505 Parnassus Avenue, San Francisco, CA 94143, USA

* Corresponding author. University of California, San Francisco, 505 Parnassus Avenue, #M551, Box 0102, San Francisco, CA 94143.

E-mail address: Arie.Perry@ucsf.edu

http://dx.doi.org/10.1016/j.path.2014.10.004
1875-9181/15/$ – see front matter © 2015 Elsevier Inc. All rights reserved.

survival among infiltrating gliomas.[3] This co-deletion is detected in approximately 80% of oligodendrogliomas, 60% of anaplastic oligodendrogliomas, 40% of oligoastrocytomas, 30% of anaplastic oligoastrocytomas, and 10% of diffuse astrocytomas of all grades. These frequencies vary considerably, however, among individual pathologists due to the subjectivity of applied morphologic criteria and contrasting philosophic biases; additionally, codeletion is rare in pediatric oligodendroglial neoplasms.[4,5] Tumors with 1p/19q codeletion almost invariably have *isocitrate dehydrogenase (IDH)* mutations.[6–8] They also frequently carry mutations in *CIC* gene on chromosome 19q and less frequently in *FUBP1* gene on chromosome 1p.[7,8] These tumors do not show *epidermal growth factor receptor (EGFR)* amplifications, which are commonly seen in primary glioblastomas, and most lack *TP53* and *alpha thalassemia/Mental retardation syndrome X-linked (ATRX)* mutations, which are common in secondary glioblastomas and lower-grade astrocytomas.[7,9,10] The combination of these multiple markers is especially useful in the differential diagnosis of anaplastic oligodendrogliomas and small cell astrocytomas, which show considerable morphologic overall but are dramatically different in terms of biological behavior.[11,12]

1p/19q codeletion is accepted as a genetic hallmark of oligodendroglial tumors and can help differentiate oligodendrogliomas from morphologically similar neoplasms, such as clear cell ependymomas, dysembryoplastic neuroepithelial tumors, and extraventricular neurocytomas.[13–15] Although a majority of these studies show nearly absolute specificity of 1p/19q codeletion for oligodendroglial tumors, it can be present in occasional extraventricular neurocytomas, representing either a unique subtype of this tumor or a true oligodendroglioma with extensive neuronal differentiation.[16,17]

Association of 1p/19q codeletion with better prognosis has been validated in multiple clinical trials.[18–20] Only recently were there sufficiently long follow-up times reported in these trials to confirm that 1p/19q codeletion is not only a prognostic but also a predictive biomarker of response to upfront chemotherapy in the setting of anaplastic oligodendroglioma.[21,22] Nevertheless, the impact of 1p/19q codeletion status on treatment recommendations varies significantly among neuro-oncologists, with some opting to postpone radiotherapy in patients with codeleted anaplastic oligodendrogliomas to reduce the risk of cognitive side effects, given the likelihood of a long survival time (average of 15 years).[23]

Data regarding the management of recurrent tumors in relation to their molecular signature are even more sparse, and utility of repeat 1p/19q testing in this setting is unclear, although one study showed that codeletion status of primary tumors and recurrences are typically identical and that 1p/19q codeletion remains a positive prognostic indicator even among recurrent tumors.[24] In addition to being rare in children, 1p/19q codeletion does not show a clear survival benefit in this cohort, where most patients do well even in the absence of such deletions.[25,26] Given that most pediatric patients with codeleted oligodendrogliomas are teenagers, it seems likely that these represent older children with adult-type gliomas.

Although various techniques, including single nucleotide polymorphism analysis and polymerase chain reaction (PCR)-based microsatellite loss of heterozygosity (LOH) and array comparative genomic hybridization (aCGH), are available to detect 1p/19q codeletion, one of the most frequent methods of detection is fluorescence in situ hybridization (FISH). Dual-color commercial probes recognizing subtelomeric regions in both arms of chromosomes 1p and 19q (1p36/1q25 and 19p13/19q13) are frequently used (**Fig. 1**). FISH can be readily applied to formalin-fixed paraffin-embedded (FFPE) tissue and does not require normal reference tissue. Although LOH studies have disadvantages in requiring normal tissue and in terms of not being morphology based, they have the advantage of being able to assess many more markers on 1p and 19q, thus providing additional clues as to whether the losses are whole arm (ie, favorable and associated with oligodendroglioma diagnosis) or smaller deletions (nonspecific). Nevertheless, there is generally high concordance between these 2 techniques and decisions regarding which one to use often rely heavily on which technique each laboratory is most comfortable implementing. Using aCGH provides even greater advantages in terms of assessing all other chromosomes for copy number alterations simultaneously, although this technique is not as widely available and is more difficult to standardize in FFPE samples.

Expression of α-internexin (INA), a neurofilament-interacting protein, was suggested as a surrogate marker of 1p/19q codeletion, with a sensitivity of 96% and a specificity of 86%.[27] Follow-up studies reported sensitivity/specificity combinations, however, of 92%/64%, 79%/80%, and 52%/85%, arguing against INA immunohistochemistry (IHC) as a sufficiently reliable technique to replace current molecular methods.[28–30]

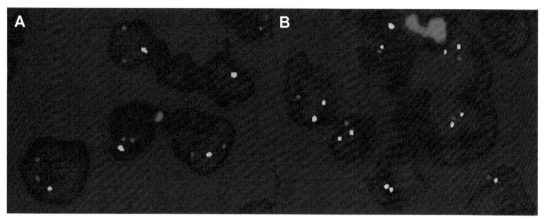

Fig. 1. FISH showing loss of 1p and 19q chromosomes: 2 red signals for 1q42 and 1 green signal for 1p32 (*A*); 2 green signals for 19p13 and 1 red signal for 19q13 (*B*).

ISOCITRATE DEHYDROGENASE GENE MUTATIONS

The IDH family encompasses 3 distinct enzymes, which are involved in the oxidative decarboxylation of isocitrate to α-ketoglutarate. IDH1 (cytoplasmic and peroxisomal) and IDH2 (mitochondrial) are homodimeric enzymes, which use NADP+ as a cofactor in this reversible reaction.[31] On the other hand, IDH3 is a mitochondrial heterodimeric enzyme, which uses NAD+ as a cofactor in an irreversible decarboxylation reaction. Deep sequencing of numerous protein-encoding regions in glioblastomas revealed mutations in *IDH* genes, which were associated with younger age and better survival.[32] Well over 90% of *IDH* mutations involve the *IDH1* gene and the remainder involve *IDH2*. The most common *IDH1* mutation is a CGT to CAT change, leading to an arginine132 to histidine substitution. This R132H form accounts for approximately 90% of all mutations.

Although 70% to 80% of grade II and III gliomas and secondary glioblastomas harbor *IDH1* or *IDI I2* gene mutations, they are rare to absent in primary glioblastomas and pilocytic astrocytomas.[33,34] *IDH* status, therefore, can help differentiate infiltrating gliomas from other glial and nonglial tumors, such as pilocytic astrocytoma, pleomorphic xanthoastrocytoma, and many low-grade tumors with oligodendroglioma-like morphology.[35–37] Similarly, *IDH* mutation provides strong support for glioblastoma with oligodendroglial component or anaplastic oligodendroglioma while essentially excluding small cell glioblastoma (SC-GBM).[38] Furthermore, the presence of *IDH* mutations can be used as a diagnostic marker of infiltrating glioma when the differential diagnosis includes gliosis or therapy-induced changes.[35,36,39,40] Nevertheless, a wild-type *IDH* result does not exclude the diagnosis of infiltrating glioma and, therefore, should not be used as evidence of gliosis in the absence of other supporting features.

In addition to important diagnostic implications, studies have reported *IDH* status as the single most powerful prognostic factor for high-grade (WHO III or IV) gliomas, being more prognostic than the histologic grade and other molecular features.[41,42] There is, however, no current difference in the treatment response between *IDH*-mutated versus *IDH* wild-type anaplastic gliomas arguing against a predictive role.[42,43] Nevertheless, the development of a targeted therapy involving the IDH pathway could change that. Prognostic and predictive roles of *IDH* mutations in low-grade (WHO II) gliomas are not as clear due to conflicting results in the literature.[44–46] Nevertheless, a recent meta-analysis supports the favorable prognostic role of *IDH* mutations among these gliomas as well.[47]

Further studies have shown that *IDH* mutations represent early events in gliomagenesis followed by *TP53* mutations or 1p/19q codeletion in astrocytic and oligodendroglial tumors, respectively.[33,48] The exact mechanism of *IDH*-induced gliomagenesis has not been established yet; however, proposed mechanisms include mutagenic effects via increased oxidative stress, angiogenesis via increased stability of hypoxia-inducible factor 1α, and epigenetic regulation via histone and DNA hypermethylation.[31] Recent findings of *IDH1* mutations being tightly related to the glioma CpG island methylator phenotype (G-CIMP) further supports its role in epigenetic regulation, with G-CIMP a direct consequence of *IDH* mutation, likely due to accumulation of the metabolite 2-hydroxyglutarate and its inhibition of DNA and histone demethylases.[49–51] The histone-methylating effect of *IDH1* mutation was implicated in the inhibition of differentiation, and selective IDH1-R132H inhibitor was shown to induce differentiation in *IDH1*-mutant glioma cell lines.[52]

IHC has been reported as a sensitive and specific method to identify tumors with *IDH1* R132H mutation using a commercially available monoclonal antibody (**Fig. 2**).[35] Although IHC does not detect *IDH2* mutations or other rare substitutions in *IDH1*, more consistent results among multiple institutions were achieved with IHC than sequencing and the sensitivity of IHC is higher because it can identify even rare individual tumor cells.[53] Sanger sequencing is an inexpensive method and is considered the gold standard for detecting *IDH* mutations. On the other hand, its sensitivity is limited to cases where mutant allele constitutes more than 20% of sample DNA; as such, false-negative results are common in low-grade gliomas with only sparse infiltrating tumor cells. Pyrosequencing was reported as an alternative and potentially more sensitive method for sequencing.[36]

EPIDERMAL GROWTH FACTOR RECEPTOR GENE ALTERATIONS

EGFR, a receptor tyrosine kinase of ERBB family (ERBB1) located on chromosome 7p12, is a strong promoter of cell proliferation and survival through its effects on mitogen-activated protein kinase and the phosphoinositol 3-kinase pathways. It has been long known that a significant portion (40%–50%) of malignant gliomas shows *EGFR* overexpression, invariably due to amplification of the *EGFR* gene.[54] Also described in gliomas are *EGFR* gene rearrangements, most commonly (20%–30%) involving the *EGFR*vIII variant characterized by in-frame deletion of exons 2–7 leading to a constitutively activated truncated receptor.[55] These *EGFR* alterations strongly suggest the diagnosis of glioblastoma, specifically the primary glioblastoma typically encountered in older patients.[56,57] *EGFR* amplification is essentially mutually exclusive with 1p/19q codeletion and *IDH* gene mutations and is identified in 70% of SC-GBMs and 40% to 50% of primary (de novo) glioblastomas in general. In combination with other alterations, such as monosomy 10, *EGFR* rearrangements represent a useful diagnostic marker to distinguish SC-GBMs from anaplastic oligodendroglioma.[11,12,58] Even in the absence of microvascular proliferation or necrosis (ie, WHO grade III on histology), such tumors have similar prognosis to glioblastomas in general when *EGFR* amplification and/or monosomy 10 are found.[11] Pilocytic astrocytomas, including clinically or histologically malignant ones, lack *EGFR* amplification, and this assay, therefore, can also be used in the critical differential diagnosis of pilocytic astrocytoma (conventional or anaplastic) and glioblastoma.[59] Combined *EGFR*/chromosome 7 centromere enumerating probe (CEP7) FISH can be used in other differential diagnosis settings to look for polysomy 7 even in the absence of *EGFR* amplification. Polysomy 7 has been detected in grade 2 astrocytomas as well as pilocytic

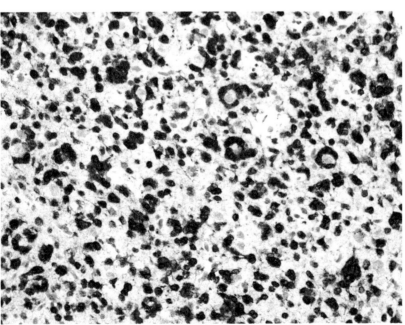

Fig. 2. IHC stain with an antibody recognizing arginine to histidine substitution at position 132 in *IDH1* shows cytoplasmic and nuclear staining in tumor cells.

astrocytomas but is absent in non-neoplastic brain tissue, suggesting an independent diagnostic role.[39,60] In addition, *EGFR* amplification is rare in pediatric high-grade gliomas whereas polysomy 7 is frequently encountered.[61–63]

Association of *EGFR* amplification with other prognostic markers causes difficulties in the assessment of its independent prognostic role. Nevertheless, some studies suggested worse outcomes in glioblastomas with *EGFR* alterations,[64] whereas others do not find a prognostic role when adjusting for the already negative prognostic effects of a glioblastoma diagnosis on histology.[65,66] Despite early recognition of *EGFR* as a target for therapy, most of the studies have failed to show treatment benefits with small molecule tyrosine kinase inhibitors.[67] Some anti-EGFRvIII vaccine trials, however, have reported promising results.[68]

EGFR amplification is detected by FISH as small fragments of extrachromosomal DNA by comparing the ratio of *EGFR/CEP7*.[69] This method, however, cannot detect *EGFR* mutations, including EGFRvIII variant. Alternative methods include chromogenic in situ hybridization and silver-enhanced in situ hybridization with similar limitations.[70,71] Endpoint or quantitative reverse transcription–PCR assays can also be used to detect both amplification and mutations. Multiplex ligation-dependent probe amplification provides a semiquantitative assay with very high specificity and sensitivity for the detection of both *EGFR* amplification and EGFRvIII.[72] IHC is a sensitive but not specific method to evaluate *EGFR* amplification because all cases of *EGFR* amplification show increased EGFR expression by IHC, but some gliomas are immunopositive due to overexpression despite a lack of gene amplification.[73,74] In addition, different clones with better sensitivity and specificity against wild-type EGFR and EGFR-vIII have been reported.[75] Unfortunately, clinical use of EGFRvIII IHC has been previously hampered by patent restrictions.

PHOSPHATASE AND TENSIN HOMOLOG DELETIONS

Phosphatase and tensin homolog (PTEN) is a tumor suppressor gene located on chromosome 10q23 encoding for an intracellular protein that inhibits phosphatidylinositol-3,4,5-triphosphate signaling, which in turn inhibits one of the gliomagenesis pathways, the AKT pathway. LOH on chromosome 10 is seen in up to 80% of both primary and secondary glioblastomas, although loss of the entire chromosome (monosomy 10) is more common in the former.[56] There are at least 3 frequently deleted loci, one of which is *PTEN*. Although *PTEN* loss in a diagnostically challenging diffuse glioma may suggest a high-grade glioma associated with poor outcome, there is no independent prognostic role of *PTEN* loss among high-grade gliomas themselves.[65,76] Studies from the temozolomide era confirms the lack of association with survival and *PTEN* loss.[77] *PTEN* loss is less frequent among high-grade pediatric gliomas; however, unlike adults, *PTEN* loss is associated with shorter survival in this setting.[62,63,78]

Loss of *PTEN* can be easily detected with commercially available probes recognizing 10q23 paired with CEP10. This method allows identification of both homozygous and hemizygous deletions of *PTEN* as well as monosomy 10.[69] Alternatively, PCR-based methods to identify LOH and IHC to identify loss of protein expression can be applied with significant correlations.[79] PTEN IHC is often difficult to interpret, however, and discordance with molecular assays is not uncommon, arguing against its routine use.[79,80]

TP53 MUTATIONS

TP53, a transcription factor and tumor suppressor gene located on chromosome 17p13, is mutated in approximately 50% of all human malignancies, leading to constitutive expression of the p53 protein.[81] Recent studies from The Cancer Genome Atlas network showed alterations involving the p53 pathway in 78% of glioblastomas.[57] These included p14(ARF) deletions, MDM2 amplification, and MDM4 amplification in addition to mutations of *TP53* itself. Other studies reported *TP53* mutations in 23% to 34% of primary glioblastomas and 60% to 79% of secondary glioblastomas.[7,9,33,56,82] The location and type of *TP53* mutations vary between primary and secondary glioblastomas, suggesting different mechanisms of acquisition. Among pediatric malignant gliomas, the rate of *TP53* mutation ranges between 12% and 40% in children younger and older than 3 years old, respectively, again suggesting different mechanisms of tumorigenesis.[83]

TP53 mutations are seen in 50% to 69% of low-grade astrocytomas, 29% to 61% of mixed oligoastrocytomas, less than 24% of oligodendrogliomas, 68% to 82% of anaplastic astrocytomas, 48% to 73% of anaplastic oligoastrocytomas, and less than 15% of anaplastic oligodendrogliomas.[7,9,10,33,48,84] Currently, p53 expression is accepted as a diagnostic biomarker, albeit a problematic one. Although the presence of *TP53* mutation or p53 overexpression strongly suggest infiltrating glioma when the differential diagnosis includes gliosis,[39] several notable exceptions of p53 positivity in non-neoplastic conditions have been published.[85] In addition, the presence of TP53 mutations suggests astrocytic rather than oligodendroglial histology, especially in the setting of intact 1p and 19q copy numbers.[33] Strong and extensive p53 immunoreactivity has similar implications but also has its exceptions.

The prognostic role of TP53 mutation is not entirely clear, and it seems related to frequency of TP53 mutation in certain histologic subtypes. TP53 mutation is associated with poor prognosis in low-grade diffuse gliomas, although the association is usually lost when controlled for astrocytic or oligodendroglial morphology.[82,86] TP53 mutations have been reported as a poor prognostic factor among primary glioblastomas,[87] whereas they seem a positive prognostic factor among secondary glioblastomas.[88] Other studies have found no prognostic or predictive value for TP53 mutations.[65,66] The p53 protein is an attractive therapeutic target due to its frequency and critical role in numerous cancers, although this is an extremely challenging pathway to target. Although still in early phases of development, novel therapies, such as virus-mediated transfection of wild-type p53 in tumors with mutant p53 and small molecule and peptide inhibitors of p53 signaling pathway, may be adopted in the treatment of glioma.[89]

CDKN2A/P16 DELETIONS

CDKN2A, a tumor suppressor gene located on chromosome 9p21 encodes p16(INK3A) and p14(ARF), which is inactivated in many cancers, including gliomas. The mechanism of inactivation is often homozygous deletion or, less commonly, hemizygous deletion with hypermethylation of the promoter region in the wild-type allele. CDKN2A deletion is seen in 30% to 68% of adult glioblastomas and 25% to 63% of anaplastic gliomas.[24,76,82,90–94] It is more frequent in de novo glioblastomas and recurrent gliomas compared with secondary glioblastomas and primary gliomas, respectively.[24,82,93] Rates for pediatric high-grade gliomas vary between 31% and 52%.[62,93] The frequency of CDKN2A loss in low-grade infiltrating gliomas are significantly lower in the literature ranging from no loss in grade II astrocytomas to 10% to 13% loss in both astrocytomas and oligodendrogliomas.[24,84,91] CDKN2A/p16 deletion is not helpful in distinguishing pilocytic astrocytomas and pleomorphic xanthoastrocytomas from infiltrating gliomas because anaplastic subsets of the former 2 also harbor deletions.[59,95] Nevertheless, the presence of homozygous CDKN2A/p16 deletion in an infiltrating glioma strongly suggests a high-grade subtype.[69]

A few studies have reported that CDKN2A loss by FISH is associated with faster progression times to higher-grade forms and shorter patient survival,[24,96] whereas others have not found an association between CDKN2A status and prognosis, especially after adjusting for histology and grade.[76,82] Similarly, studies evaluating multiple molecular markers have failed to identify a prognostic role in the management of glioblastoma.[65,66]

Although each method has advantages and disadvantages, PCR, FISH, and comparative genomic hybridization (CGH) methods can be used to detect CDKN2A deletion with high concordance rates. The PCR method is highly sensitive and specific to detect homozygous deletions when the majority of the tissue sample is composed of tumor cells; however, it may miss hemizygous deletions as well as homozygous deletions when normal tissue contamination is greater than 30%.[97] FISH can be applied on FFPE tissue and may detect most deletions. In most cases of homozygous deletion, however, 1 deletion is considerably smaller than the other; therefore, deletion may appear hemizygous or homozygous depending on the size of the smaller deletion. Additionally, cases of 2 small deletions likely will be missed. CGH is also sensitive but not widely used in FFPE samples. IHC to assess loss of p16 expression can be used with high positive predictive value for homozygous CDKN2A deletion.[93,98] Negative p16 IHC can be seen in other conditions, however, such as promoter methylation, and is not specific to CDKN2A deletion. Additionally, it can be difficult to interpret due to intermixed non-neoplastic cells. Lastly, the rates of false-positive results and false-negative results are not entirely elucidated with various commercially available antibodies.

TELOMERE MAINTENANCE MECHANISMS

Telomeres are nucleoprotein complexes at the ends of eukaryotic chromosomes, which are composed of several hundred nucleotide repeats. In the absence of telomerase, an enzyme that adds nucleotides to telomeres, telomeres progressively shorten during mitosis and telomere depletion eventually triggers cell death or senescence. Tumors may maintain their telomere length via activation of telomerase or other telomerase-independent mechanisms named as alternative lengthening of telomeres (ALT).[99] Many ALT cancers harbor mutations in ATRX or death domain–associated protein (DAXX), genes encoding proteins that interact with each other at telomeres.[100,101] Point mutations in the *telomerase reverse transcriptase* (*TERT*) gene promoter, leading to increased telomerase activity, are found in a subset of tumors, including gliomas.[102]

Recent studies indicate that gliomas can be classified based on their telomere maintenance mechanisms.[7,10,102] *TERT* promoter mutations are found in approximately 75% of oligodendrogliomas and primary glioblastomas and are significantly less frequent in WHO grade II–III astrocytomas and oligoastrocytomas.[102–104] Most gliomas lacking *TERT* promoter mutations harbor mutations of *ATRX*, and these two seem mutually exclusive.[102] *ATRX* mutations were reported in nearly 75% of WHO grade II–III astrocytomas and secondary glioblastomas.[7,9,105] Unlike their adult counterpart, pediatric glioblastomas rarely harbor *TERT* promoter mutations[104]; however, approximately 50% of the pediatric high-grade gliomas show increased telomerase activity and *hTERT* mRNA expression, suggesting other telomerase-dependent telomere maintenance mechanisms.[106] Approximately 30% of pediatric high-grade gliomas have *ATRX* mutations and ALT phenotype by FISH.[104,107]

Current data regarding the prognostic effect of *TERT* mutations are controversial, and given the strong association with *IDH* mutations, it is difficult to assess its independent role. One series reported an association with poor survival among adult primary glioblastomas,[102] whereas other series did not find a clear difference.[103] Although the former included *IDH*-mutated glioblastomas, which are almost always *TERT* wild type, the latter excluded *IDH*-mutated glioblastomas. Similarly, *TERT* mutations were associated with better survival among oligodendrogliomas, which is potentially due to its strong association with 1p/19q codeletion and *IDH* mutation.[102,103] Further complicating the matter, some studies also reported that glioblastoma patients with ALT had longer survival times, independent of age, extent of surgery, and other treatment considerations, although *IDH* mutations frequently accompanied ALT in this cohort.[108] In contrast, others found no significant associations between ALT and survival among glioblastoma patients.[109] On the other hand, among patients with "molecular astrocytomas" (gliomas without 1p19q codeletion), the presence of *ATRX* mutations was associated with better survival, independent of *IDH* status.[7,105] A recent study of pediatric high-grade gliomas failed to show prognostic significance of telomere maintenance mechanism.[106]

Although assessment of telomere maintenance mechanism may have a significant impact on molecular classification of gliomas, the best methodology to apply in a clinical setting is not entirely clear (Fig. 3). Assessment of telomerase enzyme activity and expression levels of *TERT* or other telomere-related genes requires frozen tissue and application of these to daily practice is cumbersome. Sequencing of the region of interest can identify *TERT* promoter mutations; however, this method is also not ideal for routine clinical application. The ALT phenotype can be assessed by FISH using FFPE tissue; however, its correlation with *ATRX* mutations is imperfect.[9,10,109] Similarly, a significant portion of missense mutations detected by sequencing may be missed by IHC because they would not be associated with loss of ATRX expression.[9] Furthermore, the correlation between ALT phenotype as assessed by FISH and loss of ATRX expression by IHC is also imperfect.[9,107,110] Additional studies are required to evaluate the biological significance of these various methods and their interactions with other molecular alterations.

HISTONE H3.3 MUTATIONS

Histones play critical roles in epigenetic regulation of gene expression via alterations in their post-translational modification. The human histone H3 family contains the replication-independent histone variant H3.3 in addition to canonical histones H3.1 and H3.2, which are deposited in a replication-dependent manner. Whole-exome sequencing of pediatric and adult glioblastomas revealed recurrent mutations in H3H3A, a gene that encodes the histone variant H3.3.[110] H3H3A mutations are highly specific to pediatric high-grade gliomas because they are rarely seen in other pediatric brain tumors or in adult high-grade gliomas.[110,111] Two hot spot mutations are single nucleotide variants encoding a lysine 27 to methionine (K27M) substitution, and a glycine 34 to arginine or valine (G34R/V) substitution.[110,112] Lysine 27 is one of the sites that undergoes methylation, associated with transcriptional repression, whereas glycine 34 is only 2 amino acids away from another site at lysine 36. Studies show that the H3.3 K27M mutant leads to significantly lower overall amounts of H3 with trimethylated lysine 27 (H3K27me3).[113] A later study showed that H3.3 K27M mutant gliomas lack H3K27me3 immunoreactivity, such that IHC can serve as a surrogate for molecular detection.[114]

H3H3A and *IDH* mutations are also mutually exclusive, and although the former tumors show global hypomethylation, the latter are associated with global hypermethylation (G-CIMP).[110,115] Virtually all H3.3 G34R/V mutant tumors harbor *TP53* and *ATRX/DAXX* mutations, with

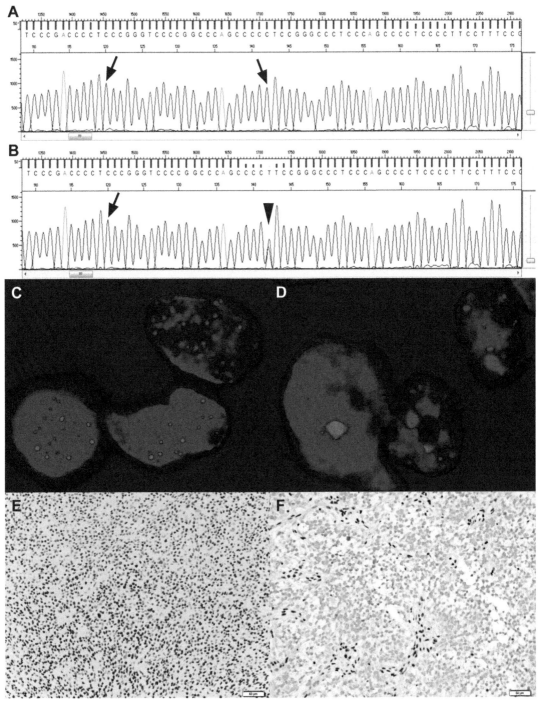

Fig. 3. Methods to assess telomere maintenance mechanisms: *TERT* promoter region by Sanger sequencing, reverse strand: wild-type (*A*) with arrows highlighting mutation hot spots at base positions 1,295,250 and 1,295,228; arrowhead highlights cytosine to thymine mutation at base position 1,295,228 (*B*). ALT phenotype by FISH: ALT-negative (*C*) and ALT-positive with large, ultrabright red telomere FISH signal (*D*). IHC stain for ATRX: nuclear expression of antibody in a tumor with wild-type *ATRX* (*E*); tumor cells with *ATRX* mutation show loss of ATRX expression whereas endothelial cells retain their expression (*F*).

hypomethylation observed most prominently in chromosome ends.[110,115] Among H3.3 K27M tumors, 60% harbor *TP53* mutations and 30% have *ATRX/DAXX* mutations.[110] Given that *ATRX/DAXX* is responsible for H3.3 deposition in pericentrometic/subtelomeric regions, it is an interesting question whether H3H3A mutations lead to genomic instability directly or act through *ATRX/DAXX* instead.

Given that H3H3A mutations are found only in pediatric high-grade gliomas, this could potentially be useful as a diagnostic marker when low-grade pediatric gliomas are in the differential.[111] Patients with H3.3 K27M tumors are typically younger than those with H3.3 G34R/V tumors.[110,115] Among high-grade gliomas, H3.3 K27M tumors are more common in midline locations, including diffuse pontine gliomas (DIPGs) and thalamic gliomas, whereas H3.3 G34R/V mutant tumors are mainly restricted to more lateral regions of the cerebral hemispheres.[110,112] This may partially explain the survival benefit of H3.3 G34R/V compared with H3.3 K27M mutant tumors.[115] Although there was no survival advantage of H3.3 K27M tumors compared with H3.3 and IDH wild-type tumors in this large cohort,[115] pediatric DIPGs with H3.3 K27M had shorter survival times than those with wild-type protein.[116]

SUMMARY

There have been major advances in the understanding of molecular characteristics of gliomas. Despite many glioma biomarkers with diagnostic, prognostic, and predictive potential identified over the past few years, advances in treatment remain limited. Although many questions remain to be answered, biomarkers, such as *IDH* and 1p/19q, are already part of routine clinical practice, whereas others will likely be added in the near future. Given the rapidity of new advances in this field, it is currently difficult to decide which tests are most critical to perform and how these results should be used for optimal patient management in the absence of large-scale prospective studies. Nevertheless, the field of molecular neuro-oncology is moving quickly, such that these questions are likely to be resolved in the near future, with an additional potential for new, targeted therapies to be developed.

REFERENCES

1. Dolecek TA, Propp JM, Stroup NE, et al. CBTRUS statistical report: primary brain and central nervous system tumors diagnosed in the United States in 2005-2009. Neuro Oncol 2012;14(Suppl 5):v1–49.

2. Louis H, Wiestler OD, Cavenee WK, editors. WHO classification of tumours of central nervous system. 4th edition. Lyon (France): IARC Press; 2007.

3. Smith JS, Perry A, Borell TJ, et al. Alterations of chromosome arms 1p and 19q as predictors of survival in oligodendrogliomas, astrocytomas, and mixed oligoastrocytomas. J Clin Oncol 2000;18:636–45.

4. Riemenschneider MJ, Jeuken JW, Wesseling P, et al. Molecular diagnostics of gliomas: state of the art. Acta Neuropathol 2010;120:567–84.

5. Kreiger PA, Okada Y, Simon S, et al. Losses of chromosomes 1p and 19q are rare in pediatric oligodendrogliomas. Acta Neuropathol 2005;109:387–92.

6. Labussiere M, Idbaih A, Wang XW, et al. All the 1p19q codeleted gliomas are mutated on IDH1 or IDH2. Neurology 2010;74:1886–90.

7. Jiao Y, Killela PJ, Reitman ZJ, et al. Frequent ATRX, CIC, FUBP1 and IDH1 mutations refine the classification of malignant gliomas. Oncotarget 2012;3:709–22.

8. Bettegowda C, Agrawal N, Jiao Y, et al. Mutations in CIC and FUBP1 contribute to human oligodendroglioma. Science 2011;333:1453–5.

9. Liu XY, Gerges N, Korshunov A, et al. Frequent ATRX mutations and loss of expression in adult diffuse astrocytic tumors carrying IDH1/IDH2 and TP53 mutations. Acta Neuropathol 2012;124:615–25.

10. Kannan K, Inagaki A, Silber J, et al. Whole-exome sequencing identifies ATRX mutation as a key molecular determinant in lower-grade glioma. Oncotarget 2012;3:1194–203.

11. Perry A, Aldape KD, George DH, et al. Small cell astrocytoma: an aggressive variant that is clinicopathologically and genetically distinct from anaplastic oligodendroglioma. Cancer 2004;101:2318–26.

12. Dehais C, Laigle-Donadey F, Marie Y, et al. Prognostic stratification of patients with anaplastic gliomas according to genetic profile. Cancer 2006;107:1891–7.

13. Fouladi M, Helton K, Dalton J, et al. Clear cell ependymoma: a clinicopathologic and radiographic analysis of 10 patients. Cancer 2003;98:2232–44.

14. Prayson RA, Castilla EA, Hartke M, et al. Chromosome 1p allelic loss by fluorescence in situ hybridization is not observed in dysembryoplastic neuroepithelial tumors. Am J Clin Pathol 2002;118:512–7.

15. Perry A, Fuller CE, Banerjee R, et al. Ancillary FISH analysis for 1p and 19q status: preliminary observations in 287 gliomas and oligodendroglioma mimics. Front Biosci 2003;8:a1–9.

16. Rodriguez FJ, Mota RA, Scheithauer BW, et al. Interphase cytogenetics for 1p19q and t(1;19)(q10;p10) may distinguish prognostically relevant subgroups in extraventricular neurocytoma. Brain Pathol 2009;19:623–9.

17. Perry A, Scheithauer BW, Macaulay RJ, et al. Oligodendrogliomas with neurocytic differentiation. A report of 4 cases with diagnostic and histogenetic implications. J Neuropathol Exp Neurol 2002;61: 947–55.

18. Cairncross JG, Ueki K, Zlatescu MC, et al. Specific genetic predictors of chemotherapeutic response and survival in patients with anaplastic oligodendrogliomas. J Natl Cancer Inst 1998;90:1473–9.

19. Cairncross G, Berkey B, Shaw E, et al. Phase III trial of chemotherapy plus radiotherapy compared with radiotherapy alone for pure and mixed anaplastic oligodendroglioma: Intergroup Radiation Therapy Oncology Group Trial 9402. J Clin Oncol 2006;24:2707–14.

20. van den Bent MJ, Carpentier AF, Brandes AA, et al. Adjuvant procarbazine, lomustine, and vincristine improves progression-free survival but not overall survival in newly diagnosed anaplastic oligodendrogliomas and oligoastrocytomas: a randomized European Organisation for Research and Treatment of Cancer phase III trial. J Clin Oncol 2006; 24:2715–22.

21. van den Bent MJ, Brandes AA, Taphoorn MJ, et al. Adjuvant procarbazine, lomustine, and vincristine chemotherapy in newly diagnosed anaplastic oligodendroglioma: long-term follow-up of EORTC brain tumor group study 26951. J Clin Oncol 2013;31:344–50.

22. Cairncross G, Wang M, Shaw E, et al. Phase III trial of chemoradiotherapy for anaplastic oligodendroglioma: long-term results of RTOG 9402. J Clin Oncol 2013;31:337–43.

23. Abrey LE, Louis DN, Paleologos N, et al. Survey of treatment recommendations for anaplastic oligodendroglioma. Neuro Oncol 2007;9:314–8.

24. Fallon KB, Palmer CA, Roth KA, et al. Prognostic value of 1p, 19q, 9p, 10q, and EGFR-FISH analyses in recurrent oligodendrogliomas. J Neuropathol Exp Neurol 2004;63:314–22.

25. Pollack IF, Finkelstein SD, Burnham J, et al. Association between chromosome 1p and 19q loss and outcome in pediatric malignant gliomas: results from the CCG-945 cohort. Pediatr Neurosurg 2003;39:114–21.

26. Raghavan R, Balani J, Perry A, et al. Pediatric oligodendrogliomas: a study of molecular alterations on 1p and 19q using fluorescence in situ hybridization. J Neuropathol Exp Neurol 2003;62: 530–7.

27. Ducray F, Criniere E, Idbaih A, et al. alpha-Internexin expression identifies 1p19q codeleted gliomas. Neurology 2009;72:156–61.

28. Eigenbrod S, Roeber S, Thon N, et al. alpha-Internexin in the diagnosis of oligodendroglial tumors and association with 1p/19q status. J Neuropathol Exp Neurol 2011;70:970–8.

29. Buckley PG, Alcock L, Heffernan J, et al. Loss of chromosome 1p/19q in oligodendroglial tumors: refinement of chromosomal critical regions and evaluation of internexin immunostaining as a surrogate marker. J Neuropathol Exp Neurol 2011;70: 177–82.

30. Nagaishi M, Suzuki A, Nobusawa S, et al. Alpha-internexin and altered CIC expression as a supportive diagnostic marker for oligodendroglial tumors with the 1p/19q co-deletion. Brain Tumor Pathol 2014;31(4):257–64.

31. Reitman ZJ, Yan H. Isocitrate dehydrogenase 1 and 2 mutations in cancer: alterations at a crossroads of cellular metabolism. J Natl Cancer Inst 2010;102:932–41.

32. Parsons DW, Jones S, Zhang X, et al. An integrated genomic analysis of human glioblastoma multiforme. Science 2008;321:1807–12.

33. Ichimura K, Pearson DM, Kocialkowski S, et al. IDH1 mutations are present in the majority of common adult gliomas but rare in primary glioblastomas. Neuro Oncol 2009;11:341–7.

34. Yan H, Parsons DW, Jin G, et al. IDH1 and IDH2 mutations in gliomas. N Engl J Med 2009;360:765–73.

35. Capper D, Weissert S, Balss J, et al. Characterization of R132H mutation-specific IDH1 antibody binding in brain tumors. Brain Pathol 2010;20: 245–54.

36. Felsberg J, Wolter M, Seul H, et al. Rapid and sensitive assessment of the IDH1 and IDH2 mutation status in cerebral gliomas based on DNA pyrosequencing. Acta Neuropathol 2010;119:501–7.

37. Capper D, Reuss D, Schittenhelm J, et al. Mutation-specific IDH1 antibody differentiates oligodendrogliomas and oligoastrocytomas from other brain tumors with oligodendroglioma-like morphology. Acta Neuropathol 2011;121:241–52.

38. Joseph NM, Phillips J, Dahiya S, et al. Diagnostic implications of IDH1-R132H and OLIG2 expression patterns in rare and challenging glioblastoma variants. Mod Pathol 2013;26:315–26.

39. Camelo-Piragua S, Jansen M, Ganguly A, et al. A sensitive and specific diagnostic panel to distinguish diffuse astrocytoma from astrocytosis: chromosome 7 gain with mutant isocitrate dehydrogenase 1 and p53. J Neuropathol Exp Neurol 2011;70:110–5.

40. Cykowski MD, Allen RA, Fung KM, et al. Pyrosequencing of IDH1 and IDH2 mutations in brain tumors and non-neoplastic conditions. Diagn Mol Pathol 2012;21:214–20.

41. Hartmann C, Hentschel B, Wick W, et al. Patients with IDH1 wild type anaplastic astrocytomas exhibit worse prognosis than IDH1-mutated glioblastomas, and IDH1 mutation status accounts for the unfavorable prognostic effect of higher age: implications for classification of gliomas. Acta Neuropathol 2010;120:707–18.

42. Wick W, Hartmann C, Engel C, et al. NOA-04 randomized phase III trial of sequential radiochemotherapy of anaplastic glioma with procarbazine, lomustine, and vincristine or temozolomide. J Clin Oncol 2009;27:5874–80.

43. van den Bent MJ, Dubbink HJ, Marie Y, et al. IDH1 and IDH2 mutations are prognostic but not predictive for outcome in anaplastic oligodendroglial tumors: a report of the European Organization for Research and Treatment of Cancer Brain Tumor Group. Clin Cancer Res 2010;16:1597–604.

44. Metellus P, Coulibaly B, Colin C, et al. Absence of IDH mutation identifies a novel radiologic and molecular subtype of WHO grade II gliomas with dismal prognosis. Acta Neuropathol 2010;120:719–29.

45. Hartmann C, Hentschel B, Tatagiba M, et al. Molecular markers in low-grade gliomas: predictive or prognostic? Clin Cancer Res 2011;17:4588–99.

46. Ahmadi R, Stockhammer F, Becker N, et al. No prognostic value of IDH1 mutations in a series of 100 WHO grade II astrocytomas. J Neurooncol 2012;109:15–22.

47. Sun H, Yin L, Li S, et al. Prognostic significance of IDH mutation in adult low-grade gliomas: a meta-analysis. J Neurooncol 2013;113:277–84.

48. Watanabe T, Nobusawa S, Kleihues P, et al. IDH1 mutations are early events in the development of astrocytomas and oligodendrogliomas. Am J Pathol 2009;174:1149–53.

49. Noushmehr H, Weisenberger DJ, Diefes K, et al. Identification of a CpG island methylator phenotype that defines a distinct subgroup of glioma. Cancer Cell 2010;17:510–22.

50. Turcan S, Rohle D, Goenka A, et al. IDH1 mutation is sufficient to establish the glioma hypermethylator phenotype. Nature 2012;483:479–83.

51. Venneti S, Thompson CB. Metabolic modulation of epigenetics in gliomas. Brain Pathol 2013;23:217–21.

52. Rohle D, Popovici-Muller J, Palaskas N, et al. An inhibitor of mutant IDH1 delays growth and promotes differentiation of glioma cells. Science 2013;340:626–30.

53. van den Bent MJ, Hartmann C, Preusser M, et al. Interlaboratory comparison of IDH mutation detection. J Neurooncol 2013;112:173–8.

54. Wong AJ, Bigner SH, Bigner DD, et al. Increased expression of the epidermal growth factor receptor gene in malignant gliomas is invariably associated with gene amplification. Proc Natl Acad Sci U S A 1987;84:6899–903.

55. Nishikawa R, Ji XD, Harmon RC, et al. A mutant epidermal growth factor receptor common in human glioma confers enhanced tumorigenicity. Proc Natl Acad Sci U S A 1994;91:7727–31.

56. Ohgaki H, Kleihues P. Genetic alterations and signaling pathways in the evolution of gliomas. Cancer Sci 2009;100:2235–41.

57. Cancer Genome Atlas Research Network. Comprehensive genomic characterization defines human glioblastoma genes and core pathways. Nature 2008;455:1061–8.

58. Korshunov A, Sycheva R, Golanov A. Molecular stratification of diagnostically challenging high-grade gliomas composed of small cells: the utility of fluorescence in situ hybridization. Clin Cancer Res 2004;10:7820–6.

59. Rodriguez EF, Scheithauer BW, Giannini C, et al. PI3K/AKT pathway alterations are associated with clinically aggressive and histologically anaplastic subsets of pilocytic astrocytoma. Acta Neuropathol 2011;121:407–20.

60. Wessels PH, Twijnstra A, Kessels AG, et al. Gain of chromosome 7, as detected by in situ hybridization, strongly correlates with shorter survival in astrocytoma grade 2. Genes Chromosomes Cancer 2002;33:279–84.

61. Bredel M, Pollack IF, Hamilton RL, et al. Epidermal growth factor receptor expression and gene amplification in high-grade non-brainstem gliomas of childhood. Clin Cancer Res 1999;5:1786–92.

62. Korshunov A, Sycheva R, Gorelyshev S, et al. Clinical utility of fluorescence in situ hybridization (FISH) in nonbrainstem glioblastomas of childhood. Mod Pathol 2005;18:1258–63.

63. Pollack IF, Hamilton RL, James CD, et al. Rarity of PTEN deletions and EGFR amplification in malignant gliomas of childhood: results from the Children's Cancer Group 945 cohort. J Neurosurg 2006;105:418–24.

64. Shinojima N, Tada K, Shiraishi S, et al. Prognostic value of epidermal growth factor receptor in patients with glioblastoma multiforme. Cancer Res 2003;63:6962–70.

65. Kraus JA, Glesmann N, Beck M, et al. Molecular analysis of the PTEN, TP53 and CDKN2A tumor suppressor genes in long-term survivors of glioblastoma multiforme. J Neurooncol 2000;48:89–94.

66. Houillier C, Lejeune J, Benouaich-Amiel A, et al. Prognostic impact of molecular markers in a series of 220 primary glioblastomas. Cancer 2006;106:2218–23.

67. van den Bent MJ, Brandes AA, Rampling R, et al. Randomized phase II trial of erlotinib versus temozolomide or carmustine in recurrent glioblastoma: EORTC brain tumor group study 26034. J Clin Oncol 2009;27:1268–74.

68. Sampson JH, Heimberger AB, Archer GE, et al. Immunologic escape after prolonged progression-free survival with epidermal growth factor receptor variant III peptide vaccination in patients with newly

diagnosed glioblastoma. J Clin Oncol 2010;28: 4722–9.

69. Horbinski C, Miller CR, Perry A. Gone FISHing: clinical lessons learned in brain tumor molecular diagnostics over the last decade. Brain Pathol 2011;21: 57–73.

70. Fischer I, de la Cruz C, Rivera AL, et al. Utility of chromogenic in situ hybridization (CISH) for detection of EGFR amplification in glioblastoma: comparison with fluorescence in situ hybridization (FISH). Diagn Mol Pathol 2008;17:227–30.

71. Gaiser T, Waha A, Moessler F, et al. Comparison of automated silver enhanced in situ hybridization and fluorescence in situ hybridization for evaluation of epidermal growth factor receptor status in human glioblastomas. Mod Pathol 2009;22: 1263–71.

72. Jeuken J, Sijben A, Alenda C, et al. Robust detection of EGFR copy number changes and EGFR variant III: technical aspects and relevance for glioma diagnostics. Brain Pathol 2009;19:661–71.

73. Viana-Pereira M, Lopes JM, Little S, et al. Analysis of EGFR overexpression, EGFR gene amplification and the EGFRvIII mutation in Portuguese high-grade gliomas. Anticancer Res 2008;28:913–20.

74. Guillaudeau A, Durand K, Pommepuy I, et al. Determination of EGFR status in gliomas: usefulness of immunohistochemistry and fluorescent in situ hybridization. Appl Immunohistochem Mol Morphol 2009;17:220–6.

75. Modjtahedi H, Khelwatty SA, Kirk RS, et al. Immunohistochemical discrimination of wild-type EGFR from EGFRvIII in fixed tumour specimens using anti-EGFR mAbs ICR9 and ICR10. Br J Cancer 2012;106:883–8.

76. Brat DJ, Seiferheld WF, Perry A, et al. Analysis of 1p, 19q, 9p, and 10q as prognostic markers for high-grade astrocytomas using fluorescence in situ hybridization on tissue microarrays from Radiation Therapy Oncology Group trials. Neuro Oncol 2004;6:96–103.

77. Carico C, Nuno M, Mukherjee D, et al. Loss of PTEN is not associated with poor survival in newly diagnosed glioblastoma patients of the temozolomide era. PLoS One 2012;7:e33684.

78. Raffel C, Frederick L, O'Fallon JR, et al. Analysis of oncogene and tumor suppressor gene alterations in pediatric malignant astrocytomas reveals reduced survival for patients with PTEN mutations. Clin Cancer Res 1999;5:4085–90.

79. Idoate MA, Soria E, Lozano MD, et al. PTEN protein expression correlates with PTEN gene molecular changes but not with VEGF expression in astrocytomas. Diagn Mol Pathol 2003;12:160–5.

80. Baeza N, Weller M, Yonekawa Y, et al. PTEN methylation and expression in glioblastomas. Acta Neuropathol 2003;106:479–85.

81. Hainaut P, Hollstein M. p53 and human cancer: the first ten thousand mutations. Adv Cancer Res 2000; 77:81–137.

82. Okamoto Y, Di Patre PL, Burkhard C, et al. Population-based study on incidence, survival rates, and genetic alterations of low-grade diffuse astrocytomas and oligodendrogliomas. Acta Neuropathol 2004;108:49–56.

83. Pollack IF, Finkelstein SD, Burnham J, et al. Age and TP53 mutation frequency in childhood malignant gliomas: results in a multi-institutional cohort. Cancer Res 2001;61:7404–7.

84. Watanabe T, Katayama Y, Yoshino A, et al. Deregulation of the TP53/p14ARF tumor suppressor pathway in low-grade diffuse astrocytomas and its influence on clinical course. Clin Cancer Res 2003;9:4884–90.

85. Kurtkaya-Yapicier O, Scheithauer BW, Hebrink D, et al. p53 in nonneoplastic central nervous system lesions: an immunohistochemical and genetic sequencing study. Neurosurgery 2002;51:1246–54 [discussion: 54–5].

86. Kim YH, Nobusawa S, Mittelbronn M, et al. Molecular classification of low-grade diffuse gliomas. Am J Pathol 2010;177:2708–14.

87. Ruano Y, Ribalta T, de Lope AR, et al. Worse outcome in primary glioblastoma multiforme with concurrent epidermal growth factor receptor and p53 alteration. Am J Clin Pathol 2009;131:257–63.

88. Li S, Zhang W, Chen B, et al. Prognostic and predictive value of p53 in low MGMT expressing glioblastoma treated with surgery, radiation and adjuvant temozolomide chemotherapy. Neurol Res 2010;32:690–4.

89. Stegh AH. Targeting the p53 signaling pathway in cancer therapy - the promises, challenges and perils. Expert Opin Ther Targets 2012;16:67–83.

90. Fan X, Munoz J, Sanko SG, et al. PTEN, DMBT1, and p16 alterations in diffusely infiltrating astrocytomas. Int J Oncol 2002;21:667–74.

91. Ueki K, Nishikawa R, Nakazato Y, et al. Correlation of histology and molecular genetic analysis of 1p, 19q, 10q, TP53, EGFR, CDK4, and CDKN2A in 91 astrocytic and oligodendroglial tumors. Clin Cancer Res 2002;8:196–201.

92. Ono Y, Tamiya T, Ichikawa T, et al. Malignant astrocytomas with homozygous CDKN2/p16 gene deletions have higher Ki-67 proliferation indices. J Neuropathol Exp Neurol 1996;55:1026–31.

93. Purkait S, Jha P, Sharma MC, et al. CDKN2A deletion in pediatric versus adult glioblastomas and predictive value of p16 immunohistochemistry. Neuropathology 2013;33:405–12.

94. Perry A, Kunz SN, Fuller CE, et al. Differential NF1, p16, and EGFR patterns by interphase cytogenetics (FISH) in malignant peripheral nerve sheath tumor (MPNST) and morphologically similar spindle

cell neoplasms. J Neuropathol Exp Neurol 2002;61: 702–9.

95. Weber RG, Hoischen A, Ehrler M, et al. Frequent loss of chromosome 9, homozygous CDKN2A/p14(ARF)/CDKN2B deletion and low TSC1 mRNA expression in pleomorphic xanthoastrocytomas. Oncogene 2007;26:1088–97.

96. Fuller CE, Schmidt RE, Roth KA, et al. Clinical utility of fluorescence in situ hybridization (FISH) in morphologically ambiguous gliomas with hybrid oligodendroglial/astrocytic features. J Neuropathol Exp Neurol 2003;62:1118–28.

97. Perry A, Nobori T, Ru N, et al. Detection of p16 gene deletions in gliomas: a comparison of fluorescence in situ hybridization (FISH) versus quantitative PCR. J Neuropathol Exp Neurol 1997;56:999–1008.

98. Rao LS, Miller DC, Newcomb EW. Correlative immunohistochemistry and molecular genetic study of the inactivation of the p16INK4A genes in astrocytomas. Diagn Mol Pathol 1997;6:115–22.

99. Bryan TM, Englezou A, Dalla-Pozza L, et al. Evidence for an alternative mechanism for maintaining telomere length in human tumors and tumor-derived cell lines. Nat Med 1997;3:1271–4.

100. Jiao Y, Shi C, Edil BH, et al. DAXX/ATRX, MEN1, and mTOR pathway genes are frequently altered in pancreatic neuroendocrine tumors. Science 2011;331:1199–203.

101. Heaphy CM, de Wilde RF, Jiao Y, et al. Altered telomeres in tumors with ATRX and DAXX mutations. Science 2011;333:425.

102. Killela PJ, Reitman ZJ, Jiao Y, et al. TERT promoter mutations occur frequently in gliomas and a subset of tumors derived from cells with low rates of self-renewal. Proc Natl Acad Sci U S A 2013;110: 6021–6.

103. Arita H, Narita Y, Fukushima S, et al. Upregulating mutations in the TERT promoter commonly occur in adult malignant gliomas and are strongly associated with total 1p19q loss. Acta Neuropathol 2013; 126:267–76.

104. Koelsche C, Sahm F, Capper D, et al. Distribution of TERT promoter mutations in pediatric and adult tumors of the nervous system. Acta Neuropathol 2013;126:907–15.

105. Wiestler B, Capper D, Holland-Letz T, et al. ATRX loss refines the classification of anaplastic gliomas and identifies a subgroup of IDH mutant astrocytic tumors with better prognosis. Acta Neuropathol 2013;126:443–51.

106. Dorris K, Sobo M, Onar-Thomas A, et al. Prognostic significance of telomere maintenance mechanisms in pediatric high-grade gliomas. J Neurooncol 2014;117:67–76.

107. Abedalthagafi M, Phillips JJ, Kim GE, et al. The alternative lengthening of telomere phenotype is significantly associated with loss of ATRX expression in high-grade pediatric and adult astrocytomas: a multi-institutional study of 214 astrocytomas. Mod Pathol 2013;26:1425–32.

108. McDonald KL, McDonnell J, Muntoni A, et al. Presence of alternative lengthening of telomeres mechanism in patients with glioblastoma identifies a less aggressive tumor type with longer survival. J Neuropathol Exp Neurol 2010;69:729–36.

109. Nguyen DN, Heaphy CM, de Wilde RF, et al. Molecular and morphologic correlates of the alternative lengthening of telomeres phenotype in high-grade astrocytomas. Brain Pathol 2013;23:237–43.

110. Schwartzentruber J, Korshunov A, Liu XY, et al. Driver mutations in histone H3.3 and chromatin remodelling genes in paediatric glioblastoma. Nature 2012;482:226–31.

111. Gielen GH, Gessi M, Hammes J, et al. H3F3A K27M mutation in pediatric CNS tumors: a marker for diffuse high-grade astrocytomas. Am J Clin Pathol 2013;139:345–9.

112. Wu G, Broniscer A, McEachron TA, et al. Somatic histone H3 alterations in pediatric diffuse intrinsic pontine gliomas and non-brainstem glioblastomas. Nat Genet 2012;44:251–3.

113. Lewis PW, Muller MM, Koletsky MS, et al. Inhibition of PRC2 activity by a gain-of-function H3 mutation found in pediatric glioblastoma. Science 2013; 340:857–61.

114. Venneti S, Garimella MT, Sullivan LM, et al. Evaluation of histone 3 lysine 27 trimethylation (H3K27me3) and enhancer of Zest 2 (EZH2) in pediatric glial and glioneuronal tumors shows decreased H3K27me3 in H3F3A K27M mutant glioblastomas. Brain Pathol 2013;23:558–64.

115. Sturm D, Witt H, Hovestadt V, et al. Hotspot mutations in H3F3A and IDH1 define distinct epigenetic and biological subgroups of glioblastoma. Cancer Cell 2012;22:425–37.

116. Khuong-Quang DA, Buczkowicz P, Rakopoulos P, et al. K27M mutation in histone H3.3 defines clinically and biologically distinct subgroups of pediatric diffuse intrinsic pontine gliomas. Acta Neuropathol 2012;124:439–47.

Practical Molecular Pathologic Diagnosis of Pilocytic Astrocytomas

Gerald F. Reis, MD, PhD, Tarik Tihan, MD, PhD*

KEYWORDS

• Pilocytic astrocytoma • Circumscribed astrocytoma • Childhood tumor

ABSTRACT

The pilocytic astrocytoma is predominantly a tumor of childhood and the most common type of circumscribed astrocytoma. The indolent nature of this tumor allows for prolonged survival for most patients, rendering the disease a rather "chronic" one, with potential long-term sequelae that are occasionally related to treatment. Two critical features of this tumor are its tendency to remain dormant, or involute even after subtotal resection, and the exceptional anaplastic transformation, sometimes following adjuvant therapy. The biological behavior of pilocytic astrocytoma can often be related to molecular alterations in the MAPK pathway.

OVERVIEW: HOW IT ALL BEGAN

The monograph by Bailey and Cushing[1] in 1926 described a cohort of cerebral and cerebellar astrocytomas that included a group of cerebellar tumors with presentation in childhood and long postoperative survival. The presence of distinct histologic features, including fibrillar and protoplasmic elements in varying proportions, was reminiscent of the entity "spongioblastoma" described by Ribbert[2] a few years earlier. Although Bailey and Cushing[1] did not distinguish the cerebral and cerebellar groups solely on the basis of histology, they noted that cerebral astrocytomas presented in adult life, were more infiltrative, less cystic, recurred early, and had a much less favorable prognosis.[3] Around the same time, Bergstrand[4] studied a similar group of cerebellar lesions from another cohort and argued that they represented hamartomas; hence, his use of the term "gliocytoma embryonale." This

interpretation, however, was not widely accepted, as illustrated by the monograph by Bucy and Gustafson,[5] which gave a formal rebuttal arguing that the hyalinized vessels, collagenized stroma, large multinucleated cells, and club-shaped or threadlike bodies represented reactive or degenerative changes within a neoplasm. In spite of being accepted by most as a neoplasm with benign behavior, the term "spongioblastoma" continued to be used for decades,[6] although Penfield and Rubinstein proposed "piloid astrocytoma" and "astrocytoma of the juvenile type," respectively.[7–10] Consensus was finally reached in 1979 when the World Health Organization (WHO) adopted the term "pilocytic astrocytoma" (PA).[11]

HOW TO INTERPRET DIFFERENT ITERATIONS OF THE WORLD HEALTH ORGANIZATION CLASSIFICATION FOR PILOCYTIC ASTROCYTOMA

PA was described in the first edition of the WHO fascicle as a neoplasm composed predominantly of fusiform cells with unusually long, wavy fibrillary processes, and frequent stellate astrocytes.[11] The cells contained nuclei with fine chromatin and unipolar or bipolar elongated processes in parallel bundles. A biphasic pattern was characteristic, with piloid areas adjacent to loose, microcystic spaces. In tumors of the posterior fossa, microcystic spaces often connected with larger cystic structures, replacing the vermis or large hemispheric portions of the cerebellum. Stromal vessels often showed hyalinized walls or endothelial proliferation, the latter being present especially in association with the cyst wall

Neuropathology Division, Department of Pathology, UCSF School of Medicine, UCSF Medical Center, 505 Parnassus Avenue, San Francisco, CA 94143-0102, USA
* Corresponding author.
E-mail address: tarik.tihan@ucsf.edu

Surgical Pathology 8 (2015) 63–71
http://dx.doi.org/10.1016/j.path.2014.10.002
1875-9181/15/$ – see front matter © 2015 Elsevier Inc. All rights reserved.

surgpath.theclinics.com

and not considered a sign of malignancy. Elongated eosinophilic, club-shaped structures (Rosenthal fibers), and eosinophilic intracytoplasmic droplets (eosinophilic granular bodies) were commonly found. These histologic features corresponded to a WHO grade I astrocytoma and encompassed cystic and solid cerebellar astrocytomas, PA of the juvenile type, and optic nerve glioma. Other characteristics included a predominantly infratentorial, posterior fossa location, with supratentorial examples typically occurring near the midline and rare cases showing large lesions in the cerebral hemisphere. Tumor growth was described as being characteristically slow, and the neoplastic cells showed only focal infiltration of the surrounding tissue. Although invasion of the subarachnoid space with moderate to marked fibroblastic leptomeningeal reaction was frequently present, this was not interpreted as a sign of malignancy. Patients were most often children and young adults, and surgical resection of tumors in the posterior fossa often resulted in cure. Anaplastic progression was seen rarely, in which case the diagnosis of anaplastic astrocytoma was suggested, histologically corresponding to WHO grade III. The "primitive polar spongioblastoma" was excluded from this category, and considered in the poorly differentiated, embryonal neoplasm category, given its malignant histology and aggressive behavior, which supported a WHO grade IV classification. The entity saw little change in the second iteration of the WHO classification.[12] Histologically, PA was defined as a slow-growing astrocytoma composed of bipolar fusiform or "piloid" cells with dense fibrillation forming compact parallel bundles and commonly showing a biphasic pattern with alternating microcystic/cystic spaces and compact areas, the latter typically containing Rosenthal fibers and eosinophilic granular bodies (Fig. 1A–C). The presence of cells with hyperchromatic and bizarre nuclei was not interpreted as a poor prognostic sign when mitotic activity was low. Immunohistochemistry for glial fibrillary acidic protein (GFAP) was always present (see Fig. 1D), but the degree of staining was noted to vary among cases. Children and young adults were primarily affected, and the peak incidence was 10 years. Many additional studies through the ensuing decade allowed for a greatly expanded discussion on PA in the third edition of the WHO classification.[13] The fundamental histologic definition and grade I designation remained the same, and more reliable information on the incidence, age and gender distribution, localization, clinical features, genetics, and prognosis was provided.[13]

This latest edition of the WHO classification scheme defines what we currently know about the clinicopathologic features of PA. The evidence supports the concept of PA as a "chronic disease" and the most common glial neoplasm affecting children.[14]

CLINICOPATHOLOGICAL PROPERTIES OF PILOCYTIC ASTROCYTOMA

The incidence of PA is estimated at 0.37 cases per 100,000 persons per year, and there is no gender predilection. Patients most often present with focal slowly progressive neurologic deficits, consistent with the tumor's indolent behavior. Initial signs can be nonlocalizing, and seizures are uncommon, yet the tumor location dictates the subsequent symptoms and signs. Although PA can arise anywhere within the central nervous system, the posterior fossa is the most common location in children and young adults. Symptoms associated with this location may include nausea, vomiting, headache, clumsiness, or gait disturbance. Patients with involvement of the optic pathway may develop vision loss and proptosis, although this may not be seen in some cases. Hypothalamic tumors can cause obesity, diabetes insipidus, obstructive hydrocephalus, and hemiparesis. Tumors of the brain stem occur in the dorsal aspect and present as an exophytic mass, sometimes extending into the cerebellopontine angle. Spinal tumors lead to nonspecific signs of cord compression.

In adults, PA generally shares common clinical manifestations with its pediatric counterpart, although some studies suggest more frequent occurrence in the cerebrum.[15–17] Symptoms associated with cerebral location are nonspecific and include generalized headaches, nausea, vomiting, visual abnormalities, and seizures. The overall mean age at diagnosis is typically between 20 and 25 years, and some series include patients diagnosed well into their 60s.[16]

RADIOLOGIC APPEARANCE OF PILOCYTIC ASTROCYTOMA

Radiologically, PA appears as a well-circumscribed, cystic mass with contrast-enhancing solid areas, commonly containing 1 or multiple cysts (Fig. 2). Optic nerve involvement is associated with nerve expansion and shows variable enhancement. The solid component is often isointense or hypointense to gray matter on T1-weighted images and hyperintense on T2-weighted images. Some PAs can be quite challenging radiologically, because they may not exhibit the classic appearance on MRI.

Fig. 1. The classic histologic features of PA include the presence of bipolar cells containing hairlike processes on cytologic preparations (*A*) (Hematoxylin & Eosin, original magnification ×400) and a biphasic appearance with alternating compact and loose areas containing microcystic spaces (*B*) (Hematoxylin & Eosin, original magnification ×100). Rosenthal fibers and eosinophilic granular bodies (*C*) (Hematoxylin & Eosin, original magnification ×400) are usually found within compact areas.

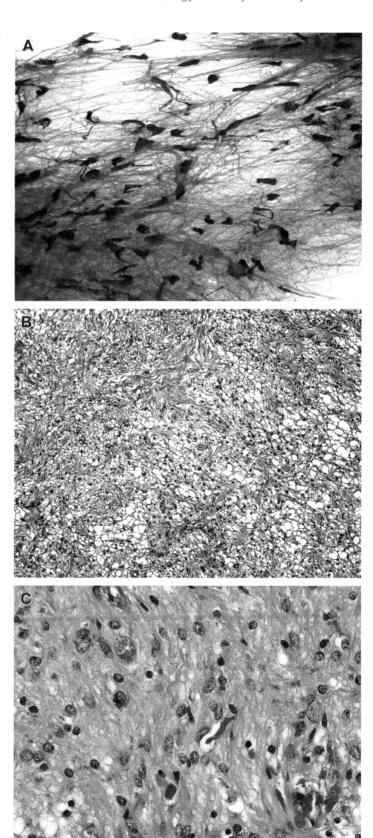

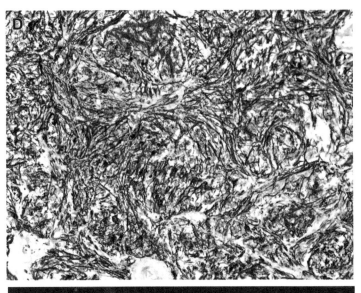

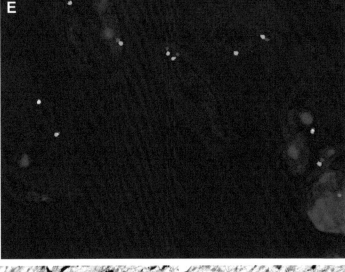

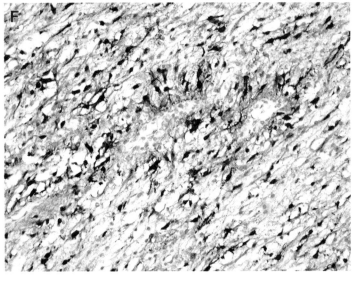

Fig. 1. (continued). The neoplasm is typically strongly and diffusely positive for GFAP (D) (Hematoxylin & Eosin, original magnification ×200). The *KIAA1549:BRAF* gene fusion is the classic molecular alteration in PA, and its presence can be detected with fluorescence in situ hybridization (E, note the yellow signal corresponding to the fusion) (Fluorescence in-situ hybridization, original magnification ×1000). In many cases, most cells show strong staining for p16 (F) (original magnification ×200), and lack of p16 staining may indicate a poor prognosis in the setting of *CDKN2A* deletion (immunohistochemical staining for p16 antigen).

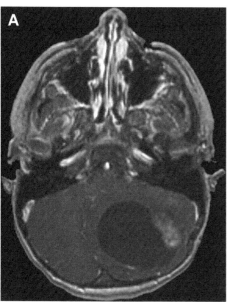 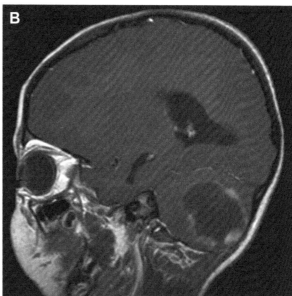

Fig. 2. Although several radiologic patterns have been described on MRI, the most common appearance of cerebral PA is that of a cystic lesion with enhancing mural nodule on T1-weighted, postgadolinium images (*A*, axial; *B*, sagittal).

THERAPY FOR PILOCYTIC ASTROCYTOMA

The therapy of choice for PA is surgical resection; however, patients with either inoperable disease or tumors not amenable to gross total resection frequently undergo chemotherapy and/or radiation.[18] Currently, chemotherapy is the preferred treatment for children younger than 10 years because of the significant adverse impact of radiotherapy on neurocognitive development.[19] Clinical trials advocate the use of combination chemotherapy with carboplatin and vincristine, given their lower toxicity in comparison with other agents and regimens, whereas radiotherapy is recommended for older children and adults with subtotal resection or tumor progression.[19–21] Nevertheless, the prognosis of PA has been reported as extremely favorable, even in cases of subtotal resection.[22] The general rule for these tumors is a protracted, indolent course. The overall survival at 5 and 10 years has been reported as 100% and 96%, respectively.[14,23] Occasional examples of spontaneous regression have been well recognized.[24,25]

Rare examples of malignant transformation may be spontaneous or show an association with radiation therapy.[26,27] Histologically, the tumors in such cases contain numerous mitoses, endothelial hyperplasia, and palisading necrosis. Interestingly, cure with or without adjuvant therapy after surgery has been reported in a subset of patients.[13] Because their prognosis has not been considered akin to glioblastoma, the 2007 WHO classification designated anaplastic (malignant) PA without a corresponding grade. It remains to be seen whether a separate grade for such anaplastic tumors is warranted.

THE AGGRESSIVE VARIANT: PILOMYXOID ASTROCYTOMA

The pilocytic category historically encompasses the pilomyxoid astrocytoma (PMA) and the "optic glioma." These deserve special consideration because the former differs from PA in a number of important ways and the latter is a nebulous term that requires a much clearer definition. PMA is composed of piloid cells and may be indistinguishable from classic PA on cytologic grounds, yet it differs histologically from PA in a number of ways. PMA typically contains a prominent myxoid matrix and monomorphous bipolar cells with angiocentric arrangement, whereas a biphasic pattern, Rosenthal fibers, and eosinophilic granular bodies are generally lacking.[28] The most common location is the hypothalamic/chiasmatic region, with less common sites including the thalamus, posterior fossa, brain stem, temporal lobe, and spinal cord.[29] Because PMA has a higher rate of recurrence and cerebrospinal fluid dissemination, WHO considers it as a grade II glial neoplasm.[13]

Optic glioma is a nonspecific clinical term, which historically has been used loosely to describe not only PA involving the optic nerve, but also infiltrating gliomas, various hypothalamic tumors, and hamartomatous lesions. Although PA is the most frequent glioma involving the optic nerve, the inclusion of other entities has led to a heterogeneous group of tumors with widely varying pathologic features and prognoses. Indeed, a growing body of evidence suggests that tumors in different locations along the optic pathway have different molecular and biological characteristics.[30] For example, unlike PMA, PA of the optic nerve has been reported to spontaneously regress even with subtotal resection or without any surgery.[31] For these reasons, it has been suggested that the term optic glioma should be avoided when referring to PA of the optic nerve.[32]

SEARCH FOR A MOLECULAR SIGNATURE AND THE DISCOVERY OF BRAF ALTERATIONS IN PILOCYTIC ASTROCYTOMA

The first recognized genetic association with PA was the NF1 gene mutation and neurofibromatosis type I (NF-1). The typical finding in these patients is bilateral optic nerve involvement.[33] Loss of NF1 was shown to activate RAS, which leads to cellular proliferation through downstream activation of the mammalian target of rapamycin pathway.[34,35] Intriguingly, PA in the setting of NF-1 was initially reported to be more indolent as compared with sporadic tumors,[36] and cases of spontaneous regression also have been reported in this setting.[25] However, subsequent studies have failed to distinguish any difference in progression-free survival or overall survival between NF-1–associated or sporadic PAs.[37]

Cytogenetic and comparative genomic hybridization studies failed to identify large chromosomal alterations promoting tumorigenesis in PA, but high-density oligonucleotide array comparative genomic hybridization analysis revealed a 1.9-MB gain at chromosome 7q34.[38–40] This alteration causes tandem duplication at 7q34 and a fusion between the KIAA1549 and BRAF genes (see **Fig. 1E**), resulting in a deletion of the amino-terminal domain of BRAF and activation of its kinase activity.[41–43] Several studies suggest that this fusion constitutes the most common molecular alteration in sporadic PA and is particularly common among posterior fossa tumors.[32,38,40,42,44–47] In addition, other molecular alterations have been reported, including additional BRAF fusion products,[48,49] rare BRAF^V600E mutations,[50] BRAF insertions,[51] and KRAS mutations.[30] It is not entirely clear to what degree each genetic alteration correlates with tumor location and behavior. Nevertheless, the biologic significance of BRAF oncogene activation lies in its ability to activate the mitogen-activated protein kinase pathway, a well-recognized early alteration in astrocytomas,[40] as well as other cutaneous and gastric neoplasms, such as melanocytic nevi and colorectal serrated polyps.[52,53]

ONCOGENE-INDUCED SENESCENCE AND ITS RELATION TO RAF/MEK/ERK PATHWAY

Oncogene-induced senescence (OIS) is a key biological mechanism controlling tumor growth and behavior. Cellular senescence refers to the process whereby proliferating cells adopt a state of permanent cell-cycle arrest.[54] Normal cells can undergo cellular senescence through oncogene overexpression, and activation of the MAPK pathway has been strongly associated with initiation of the OIS response.[54–58] The presence of BRAF oncogene alterations and MEK/MAPK activation in PA raise the possibility that these tumors also may be subjected to OIS, providing a molecular explanation for the long periods of dormancy and/or spontaneous regression.[59] Likewise, loss of NF1 leads to hyperactivation of the oncogene KRAS and downstream activation of the MAPK pathway, which can induce senescence through CDKN2A activation.[58] Indeed, immunohistochemistry for p16, the product of the CDKN2A gene, is strongly positive in PA (see **Fig. 1F**), further supporting the idea that these tumors may be subject to OIS.[32,60] Furthermore, the loss of CDKN2A in PA is associated with worse clinical outcome, suggesting that this pathway is crucial to OIS in these tumors.[60]

One caveat of using radiotherapy to treat tumors with an activated OIS may be the introduction of additional mutations or genetic silencing within crucial checkpoints, such as CDKN2A or TP53. These alterations may allow escape from senescence and increase in the aggressive behavior of tumors.[61] Indeed, earlier studies have associated anaplastic transformation of low-grade gliomas to previous radiotherapy.[26,27] Thus, therapeutic regimens that can abrogate OIS through inactivation of genes, such as CDKN2A or TP53, are more likely to be associated with a more aggressive outcome. The current evidence also confirms the historical wisdom that advises against overtreatment of such tumors.[62]

WHAT DOES THIS ALL MEAN? FUTURE DIRECTIONS

Recent studies underscore the importance of the MAPK pathway in the genesis of PA, and additional insight on OIS suggests plausible explanations for the variations in their biological behavior. Future studies are needed to identify which tumors may be subject to OIS and have the potential to regress, and which tumors may abrogate this process and act more aggressively. Understanding this biological mechanism will be crucial to the design of more effective treatment protocols for PA.

The emerging genetic diversity with respect to alterations of the MAPK pathway in PA provides a rationale for continued work toward the development of tailored therapies against targets in this pathway. The known molecular alterations in PA suggest that specific inhibitors to kinases in the MAPK pathway might provide ideal targets in the future. In fact, the results of AZD6244 (selumetinib), a MAPK inhibitor, have been modestly promising.[18] However, the complexity of the regulation of this pathway and the development of resistance to these inhibitors constitute potential limitations to single-agent therapy.[63–65] Therefore, it becomes critical to (1) determine the significance of the type of MAPK alteration in relation to treatment response (for instance, *BRAF*[V600E]-mutated tumors may benefit from therapy with vemurafenib that specifically inhibits this mutated form of *BRAF*); (2) increase the efficacy of MAPK inhibition through combination regimens; and (3) understand the critical issue of inducing or abrogating OIS depending on the choice of treatment. The availability of effective novel agents should prove useful in achieving long-term remission in cases of residual disease.

REFERENCES

1. Bailey P, Cushing H. A classification of the tumors of the glioma group on a histogenetic basis with a correlated study of prognosis. Philadelphia; London: JB Lippincott Co; 1926.

2. Ribbert H. Uber das spongioblastom und das gliom. Virchows Arch 1918;225:195–213.

3. Cushing H. Experiences with the cerebellar astrocytomas. A critical review of seventy-six cases. Surg Gynecol Obstet 1931;52:129–91.

4. Bergstrand H. Uber das sog. Astrocytom im Kleinhirn. Virchows Arch 1932;287:538–48.

5. Bucy PC, Gustafson A. Structure, nature and classification of the cerebellar astrocytomas. Am J Cancer 1939;35:327–53.

6. Ringertz N, Nordenstam H. Cerebellar astrocytoma. J Neuropathol Exp Neurol 1951;10:343–67.

7. Elvidge A, Penfield W, Cone W. The gliomas of the central nervous system: a study of two hundred and ten verified cases. Proc Assoc Res Nerv and Ment Dis 1935;16:107–81.

8. Kagan H. Anorexia and severe inanition associated with a tumour involving the hypothalamus. Arch Dis Child 1958;33:257–60.

9. Penfield W. The classification of the gliomas and neuroglial cell types. Arch Neurol Psychiatry 1931; 26:745–53.

10. Rubinstein L. Tumors of the central nervous system. 2nd edition. Bethesda (Maryland): Armed Forces Institute of Pathology; 1972.

11. Zulch KJ. 1st edition. Histologic typing of tumours of the central nervous system, vol. 21. Geneva (Switzerland): World Health Organization; 1979.

12. Kleihues P, Burger PC, Scheithauer BW. Histologic typing of tumours of the central nervous system. 2nd edition. Berlin: Springer-Verlag Berlin Heidelberg; 1993.

13. Scheithauer BW, Hawkins C, Tihan T, et al. In: Louis D, Ohgaki H, Wiestler OD, et al, editors. WHO Classification of Tumours of the Central Nervous System. Pilocytic astrocytoma. 4th edition. Lyon (France): International Agency for Research on Cancer; 2007. p. 14–21.

14. Ohgaki H, Kleihues P. Population-based studies on incidence, survival rates, and genetic alterations in astrocytic and oligodendroglial gliomas. J Neuropathol Exp Neurol 2005;64:479–89.

15. Clark GB, Henry JM, McKeever PE. Cerebral pilocytic astrocytoma. Cancer 1985;56:1128–33.

16. Forsyth PA, Shaw EG, Scheithauer BW, et al. Supratentorial pilocytic astrocytomas. A clinicopathologic, prognostic, and flow cytometric study of 51 patients. Cancer 1993;72:1335–42.

17. Garcia DM, Fulling KH. Juvenile pilocytic astrocytoma of the cerebrum in adults. A distinctive neoplasm with favorable prognosis. J Neurosurg 1985;63:382–6.

18. Sadighi Z, Slopis J. Pilocytic astrocytoma: a disease with evolving molecular heterogeneity. J Child Neurol 2013;28:625–32.

19. Perilongo G. Considerations on the role of chemotherapy and modern radiotherapy in the treatment of childhood low grade glioma. J Neurooncol 2005; 75:301–7.

20. Ater JL, Zhou T, Holmes E, et al. Randomized study of two chemotherapy regimens for treatment of low-grade glioma in young children: a report from the Children's Oncology Group. J Clin Oncol 2012;30:2641–7.

21. Packer RJ, Ater J, Allen J, et al. Carboplatin and vincristine chemotherapy for children with newly diagnosed progressive low-grade gliomas. J Neurosurg 1997;86:747–54.

22. Fisher PG, Breiter SN, Carson BS, et al. A clinicopathologic reappraisal of brain stem tumor classification. Identification of pilocystic astrocytoma and fibrillary astrocytoma as distinct entities. Cancer 2000;89:1569–76.

23. Fernandez C, Figarella-Branger D, Girard N, et al. Pilocytic astrocytomas in children: prognostic

factors–a retrospective study of 80 cases. Neurosurgery 2003;53:544–53 [discussion: 554–5].

24. Gunny RS, Hayward RD, Phipps KP, et al. Spontaneous regression of residual low-grade cerebellar pilocytic astrocytomas in children. Pediatr Radiol 2005;35:1086–91.

25. Legius E, Marchuk DA, Collins FS, et al. Somatic deletion of the neurofibromatosis type 1 gene in a neurofibrosarcoma supports a tumour suppressor gene hypothesis. Nat Genet 1993;3:122–6.

26. Dirks PB, Jay V, Becker LE, et al. Development of anaplastic changes in low-grade astrocytomas of childhood. Neurosurgery 1994;34:68–78.

27. Tomlinson FH, Scheithauer BW, Hayostek CJ, et al. The significance of atypia and histologic malignancy in pilocytic astrocytoma of the cerebellum: a clinicopathologic and flow cytometric study. J Child Neurol 1994;9:301–10.

28. Tihan T, Fisher PG, Kepner JL, et al. Pediatric astrocytomas with monomorphous pilomyxoid features and a less favorable outcome. J Neuropathol Exp Neurol 1999;58:1061–8.

29. Komotar RJ, Mocco J, Carson BS, et al. Pilomyxoid astrocytoma: a review. MedGenMed 2004;6:42.

30. Forshew T, Tatevossian RG, Lawson AR, et al. Activation of the ERK/MAPK pathway: a signature genetic defect in posterior fossa pilocytic astrocytomas. J Pathol 2009;218:172–81.

31. Parsa CF, Hoyt CS, Lesser RL, et al. Spontaneous regression of optic gliomas: thirteen cases documented by serial neuroimaging. Arch Ophthalmol 2001;119:516–29.

32. Reis GF, Bloomer MM, Perry A, et al. Pilocytic astrocytomas of the optic nerve and their relation to pilocytic astrocytomas elsewhere in the central nervous system. Mod Pathol 2013;26:1279–87.

33. Lewis RA, Gerson LP, Axelson KA, et al. von Recklinghausen neurofibromatosis. II. Incidence of optic gliomata. Ophthalmology 1984;91:929–35.

34. Chen YH, Gutmann DH. The molecular and cell biology of pediatric low-grade gliomas. Oncogene 2014;33:2019–26.

35. Dasgupta B, Yi Y, Chen DY, et al. Proteomic analysis reveals hyperactivation of the mammalian target of rapamycin pathway in neurofibromatosis 1-associated human and mouse brain tumors. Cancer Res 2005;65:2755–60.

36. Rorke LB, Packer RJ, Biegel JA. Central nervous system atypical teratoid/rhabdoid tumors of infancy and childhood: definition of an entity. J Neurosurg 1996;85:56–65.

37. Tihan T, Ersen A, Qaddoumi I, et al. Pathologic characteristics of pediatric intracranial pilocytic astrocytomas and their impact on outcome in 3 countries: a multi-institutional study. Am J Surg Pathol 2012;36:43–55.

38. Bar EE, Lin A, Tihan T, et al. Frequent gains at chromosome 7q34 involving BRAF in pilocytic astrocytoma. J Neuropathol Exp Neurol 2008;67:878–87.

39. Deshmukh H, Yeh TH, Yu J, et al. High-resolution, dual-platform aCGH analysis reveals frequent HIPK2 amplification and increased expression in pilocytic astrocytomas. Oncogene 2008;27:4745–51.

40. Pfister S, Janzarik WG, Remke M, et al. BRAF gene duplication constitutes a mechanism of MAPK pathway activation in low-grade astrocytomas. J Clin Invest 2008;118:1739–49.

41. Ciampi R, Knauf JA, Kerler R, et al. Oncogenic AKAP9-BRAF fusion is a novel mechanism of MAPK pathway activation in thyroid cancer. J Clin Invest 2005;115:94–101.

42. Jones DT, Kocialkowski S, Liu L, et al. Tandem duplication producing a novel oncogenic BRAF fusion gene defines the majority of pilocytic astrocytomas. Cancer Res 2008;68:8673–7.

43. Tran NH, Wu X, Frost JA. B-Raf and Raf-1 are regulated by distinct autoregulatory mechanisms. J Biol Chem 2005;280:16244–53.

44. Jacob K, Albrecht S, Sollier C, et al. Duplication of 7q34 is specific to juvenile pilocytic astrocytomas and a hallmark of cerebellar and optic pathway tumours. Br J Cancer 2009;101:722–33.

45. Rodriguez FJ, Ligon AH, Horkayne-Szakaly I, et al. BRAF duplications and MAPK pathway activation are frequent in gliomas of the optic nerve proper. J Neuropathol Exp Neurol 2012;71:789–94.

46. Sievert AJ, Jackson EM, Gai X, et al. Duplication of 7q34 in pediatric low-grade astrocytomas detected by high-density single-nucleotide polymorphism-based genotype arrays results in a novel BRAF fusion gene. Brain Pathol 2009;19:449–58.

47. Yu J, Deshmukh H, Gutmann RJ, et al. Alterations of BRAF and HIPK2 loci predominate in sporadic pilocytic astrocytoma. Neurology 2009;73:1526–31.

48. Cin H, Meyer C, Herr R, et al. Oncogenic FAM131B-BRAF fusion resulting from 7q34 deletion comprises an alternative mechanism of MAPK pathway activation in pilocytic astrocytoma. Acta Neuropathol 2011;121:763–74.

49. Jones DT, Kocialkowski S, Liu L, et al. Oncogenic RAF1 rearrangement and a novel BRAF mutation as alternatives to KIAA1549:BRAF fusion in activating the MAPK pathway in pilocytic astrocytoma. Oncogene 2009;28:2119–23.

50. Schindler G, Capper D, Meyer J, et al. Analysis of BRAF V600E mutation in 1,320 nervous system tumors reveals high mutation frequencies in pleomorphic xanthoastrocytoma, ganglioglioma and extra-cerebellar pilocytic astrocytoma. Acta Neuropathol 2011;121:397–405.

51. Eisenhardt AE, Olbrich H, Roring M, et al. Functional characterization of a BRAF insertion mutant associated with pilocytic astrocytoma. Int J Cancer 2011;129:2297–303.

52. Kuilman T, Michaloglou C, Mooi WJ, et al. The essence of senescence. Genes Dev 2010;24:2463–79.

53. Minoo P, Jass JR. Senescence and serration: a new twist to an old tale. J Pathol 2006;210:137–40.

54. Campisi J, d'Adda di Fagagna F. Cellular senescence: when bad things happen to good cells. Nat Rev Mol Cell Biol 2007;8:729–40.

55. Cagnol S, Chambard JC. ERK and cell death: mechanisms of ERK-induced cell death–apoptosis, autophagy and senescence. FEBS J 2010;277:2–21.

56. Evan GI, d'Adda di Fagagna F. Cellular senescence: hot or what? Curr Opin Genet Dev 2009;19:25–31.

57. Lin AW, Barradas M, Stone JC, et al. Premature senescence involving p53 and p16 is activated in response to constitutive MEK/MAPK mitogenic signaling. Genes Dev 1998;12:3008–19.

58. Serrano M, Lin AW, McCurrach ME, et al. Oncogenic ras provokes premature cell senescence associated with accumulation of p53 and p16INK4a. Cell 1997; 88:593–602.

59. Borit A, Richardson EP Jr. The biological and clinical behaviour of pilocytic astrocytomas of the optic pathways. Brain 1982;105:161–87.

60. Raabe EH, Lim KS, Kim JM, et al. BRAF activation induces transformation and then senescence in human neural stem cells: a pilocytic astrocytoma model. Clin Cancer Res 2011;17:3590–9.

61. Horbinski C, Nikiforova MN, Hagenkord JM, et al. Interplay among BRAF, p16, p53, and MIB1 in pediatric low-grade gliomas. Neuro Oncol 2012;14: 777–89.

62. Burger PC, Scheithauer BW, Lee RR, et al. An interdisciplinary approach to avoid the overtreatment of patients with central nervous system lesions. Cancer 1997;80:2040–6.

63. Emery CM, Vijayendran KG, Zipser MC, et al. MEK1 mutations confer resistance to MEK and B-RAF inhibition. Proc Natl Acad Sci U S A 2009;106:20411–6.

64. Kolb EA, Gorlick R, Houghton PJ, et al. Initial testing (stage 1) of AZD6244 (ARRY-142886) by the Pediatric Preclinical Testing Program. Pediatr Blood Cancer 2010;55:668–77.

65. Wee S, Jagani Z, Xiang KX, et al. PI3K pathway activation mediates resistance to MEK inhibitors in KRAS mutant cancers. Cancer Res 2009;69: 4286–93.

Practical Molecular Pathology and Histopathology of Embryonal Tumors

Joanna Phillips, MD, PhD[a],*, Tarik Tihan, MD, PhD[a],
Gregory Fuller, MD, PhD[a,b]

KEYWORDS

- Embryonal tumors • Molecular pathology • Histopathology • WHO classification

ABSTRACT

There have been significant improvements in understanding of embryonal tumors of the central nervous system (CNS) in recent years. These advances are most likely to influence the diagnostic algorithms and methodology currently proposed by the World Health Organization (WHO) classification scheme. Molecular evidence suggests that the tumors presumed to be specific entities within the CNS/primitive neuroectodermal tumors spectrum are likely to be reclassified. All these developments compel reassessing current status and expectations from the upcoming WHO classification efforts. This review provides a synopsis of current developments and a practical algorithm for the work-up of these tumors in practice.

EMBRYONAL TUMORS IN WORLD HEALTH ORGANIZATION CLASSIFICATION

The original works of Cushing and Bailey were the first systematic efforts in the classification of tumors of the central nervous system (CNS).[1,2] In these seminal attempts, these investigators provided a rational and clinically relevant classification of intracranial tumors. Both investigators, together and separately, have incorporated an embryonal cell of origin hypothesis and provided the first nomenclature of embryonal, or blastic, tumors that has prevailed until present day.[3,4] In neither of the initial classification attempts of this school

did embryonal tumors constitute a distinct category but were distributed among various categories of the scheme. The subsequent attempts, including the first classification of the World Health Organization (WHO), began segregating tumors into the "poorly differentiated and embryonal tumors" category.[5,6] This version of the classification scheme included glioblastoma and medulloblastoma within the same category of tumors.[2,5] After the publication of the first edition of the WHO, ensuing efforts in 1988 and 1990 led to a second classification attempt in 1993, in which the tumor grouping included morphology codes of the *International Classification of Diseases for Oncology* and the Systematized Nomenclature of Medicine for the first time.[7] This classification attempt clearly distinguished the embryonal tumor category from the glial and neuronal tumors as well as pineal parenchymal tumors, including pineoblastoma.

The classifications in 2000 and 2007 further refined the paradigms adopted in the 1993 edition and presented data for additional distinct entities.[1,8] Atypical teratoid/rhabdoid tumor (AT/RT) and large cell/anaplastic medulloblastoma (LC/A) were added in 2000, and the CNS primitive neuroectodermal tumors (PNETs) group was added in 2007.[1,8] The latter category included a group of tumor types, such as ganglioneuroblastoma, neuroblastoma, medulloepithelioma, and ependymoblastoma, that were considered distinct entities in 2000. The 2007 classification also included the CNS prefix to the PNETs category to enable a

[a] Neuropathology Division, Department of Pathology, UCSF School of Medicine, UCSF Medical Center, Room M551, 505 Parnassus Avenue, San Francisco, CA, USA; [b] University of Texas MD Anderson Cancer Center, Houston, TX, USA
* Corresponding author.
E-mail address: joanna.phillips@ucsf.edu

Surgical Pathology 8 (2015) 73–88
http://dx.doi.org/10.1016/j.path.2014.10.003

clear distinction from the tumors with the same name that occur at extracerebral sites.

Much has evolved since the publication of the last WHO classification scheme, and the additional information and insight gained during this period have affected almost all the entities in the embryonal tumor category. This article briefly summarizes these advances and the probable changes in the upcoming revision of the classification scheme.

MEDULLOBLASTOMAS

Medulloblastoma is the most common pediatric malignant brain tumor. This embryonal neoplasm of the cerebellum can be subdivided into several histopathologic variants according to the 2007 WHO classification scheme.[1] These variants include

- Classic medulloblastoma
- Desmoplastic/nodular medulloblastoma
- Medulloblastoma with extensive nodularity (MBEN)
- Anaplastic medulloblastoma
- Large cell medulloblastoma

Although medulloblastoma is a highly malignant tumor, classified as WHO grade IV, LC/As tend to be associated with a significantly worse prognosis and have a higher frequency of metastatic disease than other medulloblastomas.[9–11] With current therapeutic management, including surgical resection, craniospinal radiation, and chemotherapy, a majority of patients can be cured of their tumor, even though most have long-term disabilities.[12–14] These disabilities can be attributed to both their underlying disease and to the treatment.

RISK STRATIFICATION AND PROGNOSTICATION FOR MEDULLOBLASTOMAS

Because therapy is not benign, risk stratification is essential. Currently, risk stratification is based on histologic subgroup and clinical variables. Tumors with leptomeningeal metastases and incomplete surgical resection confer a higher risk. In addition, specific molecular alterations have been associated with poor prognosis, including isochromosome 17q, loss of 17p, and amplification of *MYC* or *MYCN*.[11,15,16] Similarly, nuclear accumulation of β-catenin (indicative of canonical WNT pathway activation) and monosomy 6 have been associated with a better prognosis.[11,17] Despite these advances, accurate assessment of disease risk for individual patients can be difficult.

Several researchers have used molecular strategies, including transcriptional profiling, to improve disease prognostication and stratification into molecular subgroups. In 2010, a consensus conference was held in which 4 subgroups of medulloblastoma were defined with unique demographic, clinical, transcriptional, and genetic differences.[18] Later, in 2013, a meeting of the International Medulloblastoma Working Group[19] recommended that the WHO classification of medulloblastoma be revised to incorporate both histopathologic and molecular categorization.

Because the histopathologic variants fit within more than 1 molecular subgroup, this discussion begins with the characteristic features of the 4 well-known histopathologic variants.[1,20] Many studies have helped define characteristic demographic, clinical, and molecular features of these subtypes, refining their prognostic implications. Then, the molecular subgroups are focused on, summarizing their demographic and clinical differences and the histopathologic variants they encompass. The currently accepted variants within the entity of medulloblastoma are briefly defined.

CLASSIC MEDULLOBLASTOMA

The classic variant is the most common and is characterized by a highly cellular, typically patternless neoplasm composed of highly proliferative cells with small to medium-sized nuclei, relatively unapparent nucleoli, nuclear molding, and minimal cytoplasm (**Fig. 1**A). Necrosis and karyorrhexis are common. As with all medulloblastomas, neuronal differentiation may be observed and can be highlighted by immunohistochemistry.

VARIANT: DESMOPLASTIC/NODULAR MEDULLOBLASTOMA

The desmoplastic/nodular variant is defined by striking nodules of differentiation resulting in reticulin-poor intranodular foci surrounded by densely cellular, proliferative reticulin-rich internodular regions (see **Fig. 1**B). These tumors are most often located in the lateral cerebellar hemispheres in patients ages 3 to 16 years. They are often located laterally within the hemispheres (see **Fig. 1**C) unlike the WNT group (group 1) tumors that are located in the midline.

VARIANT: MEDULLOBLASTOMA WITH EXTENSIVE NODULARITY

MBEN is largely composed of the reticulin-free pale areas and is most common in infants. MBEN has typical radiologic features with multiple nodules, often referred to as a bunch of grapes appearance (see **Fig. 1**D).

Fig. 1. (*A*) Classical variant of medulloblastoma on routine H&E stains, demonstrating small, blue, round cell morphology and numerous Homer Wright rosettes (original magnification, ×200). (*B*) Typical histologic appearance of MBEN on low-power images. The tumor is composed of predominantly well differentiated nodules with paucicellularity, also known as pale islands, surrounded by fibrous septations and hypercellular internodular areas (original magnification, ×40).

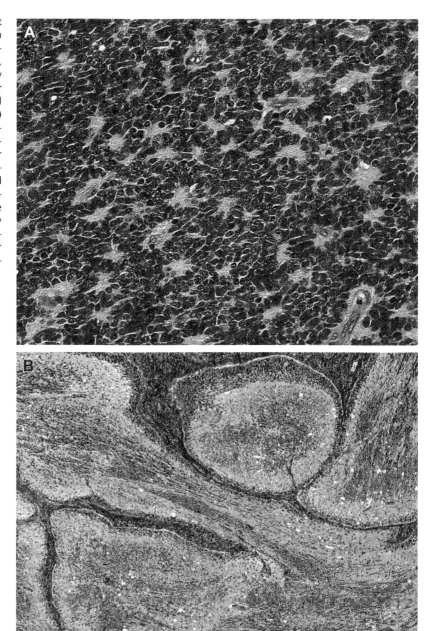

VARIANT(S): LARGE CELL AND ANAPLASTIC MEDULLOBLASTOMA

LC/A represents the combination of 2 morphologic patterns, both with poor prognosis and both considered as variants. The large cell variant is characterized by large, vesicular nuclei and prominent nucleoli (see Fig. 1E). Increased nuclear size, atypical mitotic forms, abundant apoptotic bodies, and cell wrapping characterize the anaplastic variant (see Fig. 1F).

Other less common subtypes include medulloblastoma with myogenic or melanocytic differentiation. The latter 2 are currently considered patterns other than distinct variants.

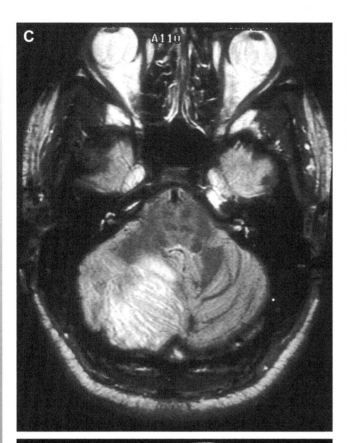

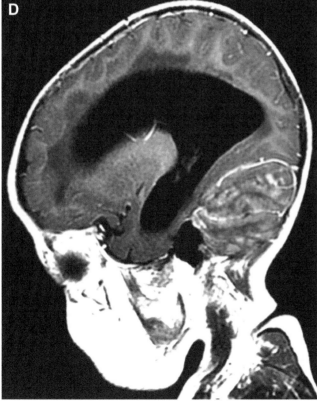

Fig. 1. (*continued*). (*C*) Radiologic appearance of desmoplastic/nodular medulloblastoma on axial T2-based imaging, showing a peripheric involvement and expansion of the right cerebellar hemisphere. (*D*) Radiologic appearance of desmoplastic MBEN on sagittal contrast-enhanced T1-weighted imaging demonstrating a multinodular, bunch of grapes–like appearance and associated hydrocephalus.

Fig. 1. (continued). (E) High-power magnification of the large cell variant demonstrating discohesive, large cell lymphoma–like anaplastic cells with prominent nucleoli and numerous mitotic and apoptotic cells (original magnification, ×400). *(F)* High-power magnification of the anaplastic variant showing hyperchromatic enlarged nuclei with marked pleomorphism suggesting anaplastic histologic pattern (original magnification, ×400).

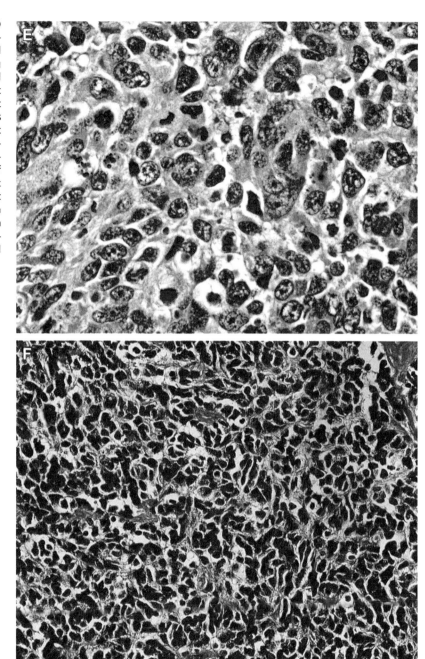

CLASSIFICATION OF MEDULLOBLASTOMA BASED ON MOLECULAR CRITERIA

Based on molecular criteria, currently proposed subgroups of medulloblastoma are[18,19]

1. WNT (Group 1)
2. SHH (Group 2)
3. Non-WNT/Non-SHH (Group 3)
4. Non-WNT/Non-SHH (Group 4)

WNT Pathway Tumors (Molecular Group 1)

As suggested by the name, the WNT subgroup is characterized by expression of WNT signaling pathway genes. These tumors are almost exclusively of the classic morphology. The tumor can be seen in both children and adults, metastases are rare, and overall prognosis is good. Some WNT medulloblastomas with LC/A morphology have been reported, and they seem to have a better prognosis than might be expected based on their histology.[21] WNT subgroup tumors typically demonstrate nuclear immunopositivity for β-catenin (**Fig. 2**A), mutations in CTNNB1, mutations in DDX3X, and monosomy 6.[18] WNT tumors also have characteristic methylation profiling and gene expression patterns. Abnormal WNT signaling may be particularly important in driving these tumors, and data from model systems suggest transformation of neural progenitor cell populations in the lower rhombic lip of the dorsal brainstem may be particularly important in this subtype.[22]

Sonic Hedgehog (SHH) Pathway Tumors (Molecular Group 2)

The SHH subgroup includes tumors thought to be driven by the Sonic Hedgehog signaling pathway. This subgroup encompasses most desmoplastic/nodular medulloblastomas, including MBEN, but

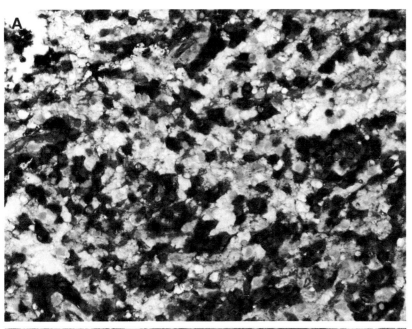

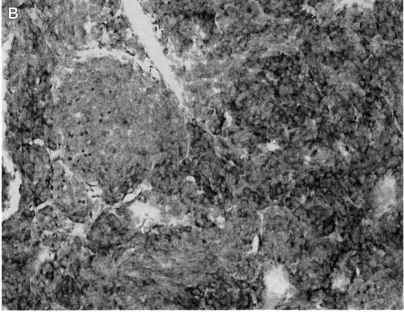

Fig. 2. (A) High-power magnification image of immunohistochemical staining with the β-catenin antibody. The interpretation of this stain can be challenging because the significant staining is actually the nuclear positivity and the cytoplasmic positivity should be ignored in terms of WNT pathway activation (original magnification, ×400). (B) Immunohistochemical staining with the GAB1 antibody, which is essentially cytoplasmic (original magnification, ×200).

it also includes a significant subset of classic and LC/A tumors. Patients with this subtype include infants (age 0–3 years) and adults (age >16 years) and overall prognosis is intermediate between that of WNT tumors and group 3 tumors. Characterized by a unique methylation profiling pattern and gene expression pattern, these tumors are also frequently immunopositive for GAB1 (see Fig. 2B) and harbor mutations in the SHH signaling pathway genes, including deletion of chromosome 9q that contains the PTCH gene.[23] Unlike the WNT tumors, SHH tumors may arise from granule neuron precursors in the cerebellum. During normal development, Purkinje cells secrete SHH to promote the proliferation of external granule neurons. Therapeutics targeting the SHH pathway may be particularly effective in this subgroup of medulloblastoma.

Non-WNT/Non-SHH Pathway Tumors (Molecular Groups 3 and 4)

Unlike in the WNT and SHH subtypes, the underlying drivers for the group 3 and group 4 tumors are not yet clear and these are sometimes referred to as the non-WNT/non-SHH subgroup. Group 3 and group 4 tumors, however, have unique methylation profiles, patterns of gene expression, and prognosis. Group 3 tumors, most common in male patients, have the worst prognosis and are frequently metastatic at diagnosis. The previous association of metastatic disease with poor prognosis may be due to the enrichment of group 3 tumors in this clinical subset.[23] Group 3 tumors also commonly exhibit high MYC expression levels and MYC amplification (but not NMYC amplification)[23,24] and they often occur in infants or children. It has been suggested that MYC amplification may identify a particularly aggressive subset within this tumor subgroup.[25] Although a majority of group 3 tumors have classic histology, most LC/As belong to this subgroup. In contrast, the group 4 medulloblastomas have an intermediate prognosis that is more similar to the SHH tumors. In general, this subgroup is more common in male patients and is associated with isochromosome 17q. Group 4 tumors are associated with loss of the X chromosome, and they encompass both classic and large cell/anaplastic variants.

Although medulloblastoma molecular subtypes improve risk stratification, there is still debate as to how these subtypes should be defined clinically. Gene expression analysis using the NanoString platform has been shown a robust method to determine tumor subtype using formalin-fixed paraffin-embedded (FFPE) tumor

tissues from around the world.[23] Studies have also demonstrated robust molecular stratification of FFPE tumor tissues by methylation profiling using the Illumina GoldenGate DNA methylation array or the Infinium HumanMethylation450 BeadChip array.[26,27] In addition, immunohistochemistry-based strategies have been reported that can easily be applied by most pathology laboratories[21,24]; however, due to reported overlap between subtypes, additional markers or complementary methods may be needed.[27] Regardless of the method, molecular subtyping improves disease prognostication in medulloblastoma. Moreover, many groups are already beginning to refine the granularity of the molecular subtypes and trying to identify prognostic biomarkers within each molecular subtype.[25]

In summary, the practical work-up of medulloblastomas in the pathology laboratory should include immunohistochemical stains for β-catenin, GAB-1, and fluorescence in situ hybridization analyses for MYC and NMYC as well as isochromosome 17q. It will be possible to determine the validity of high throughput genetic analysis in the near future.

ATYPICAL TERATOID/RHABDOID TUMOR AND OTHER MALIGNANT RHABDOID TUMORS IN THE CENTRAL NERVOUS SYSTEM

AT/RT is a malignant CNS neoplasm with a strong propensity of arising during infancy and early childhood (first 3 years of life), although it also affects the adult population.[28] The awkward name reflects the fact that tumors falling at the 2 ends of the morphologic spectrum, "pure" CNS rhabdoid tumor and malignant teratoid tumor, were not initially recognized as part of the same family, the definitive proof of which was provided by demonstration of a common molecular signature, namely loss or mutation of the SMARCB1 (INI1, hSNF5, BAF47) gene on chromosome 22.[29] In the pediatric population, approximately 60% of tumors arise in the posterior fossa (cerebellum, cerebellopontine angle) and 40% in the cerebrum (Fig. 3A). In older patients, AT/RT is also well documented in unusual locations, such as the pineal gland and sellar region, in addition to its usual posterior fossa or cerebral location.[30]

Although the name implies that rhabdoid morphology is an integral feature of AT/RT, such is not the case in a majority of examples. Rather, AT/RT typically is composed of a heterogeneous mixture of cellular elements, with large pale

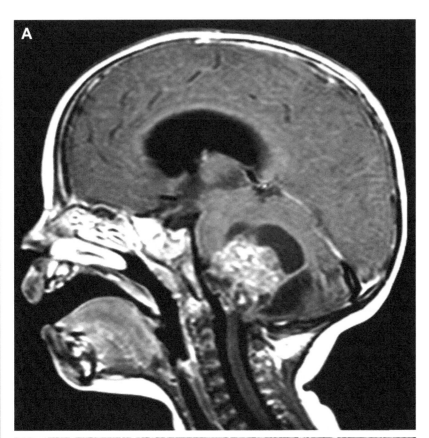

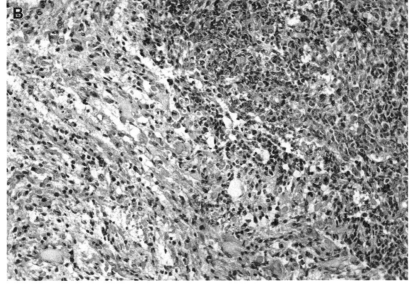

Fig. 3. (A) Sagittal contrast-enhanced T1-weighted image of an infant with an AT/RT involving the posterior fossa and associated hydrocephalus. (B) Histologic appearance of both the PNET-like (upper left) and the bland, large cells (lower right) of AT/RT (original magnification, ×200).

Fig. 3. (continued). (C) Rhabdoid cells admixed with small, primitive cells in AT/RT (original magnification, ×400). (*D*) Immunohistochemical staining for EMA antibody in AT/RT (original magnification, ×400).

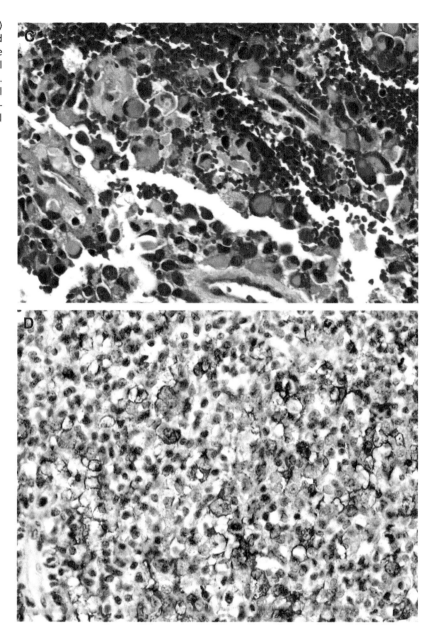

cells figuring prominently in most tumors, with small PNET-like rhabdoid and epithelial components variably represented (see **Fig. 3**B, C). This heterogeneity is typically also reflected immunohistochemically in a polyphenotypic profile, with epithelial membrane antigen (EMA) and smooth muscle actin (SMA) expression present focally in approximately 95% and 75% of cases, respectively (see **Fig. 3**D, E), and other differentiation markers, such as synaptophysin and glial fibrillary acidic protein (GFAP), variably present from case-to-case.[31] The diagnosis of AT/RT is confirmed by demonstration of INI loss through immunostaining (see **Fig. 3**F) or molecular methods. Because the morphologic spectrum of AT/RT as seen on hematoxylin-eosin (H&E)-stained tissue sections can overlap significantly with that of medulloblastoma, INI1 testing (typically by immunohistochemistry) of all posterior fossa PNETs has become a routine procedure

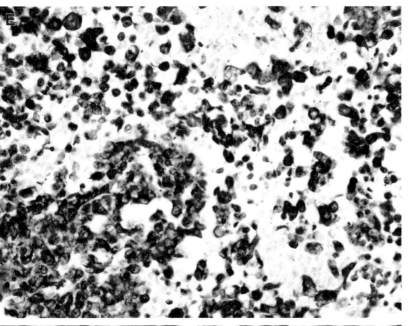

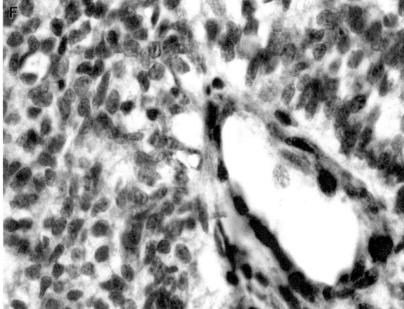

Fig.   3. (continued). (E) Immunohistochemical staining with the SMA antibody in ATRT (original   magnification, ×400). (F) BAF-47 staining in AT/RT demonstrating loss of nuclear staining suggestive of a loss of function mutation in SMARCB1 gene. The vascular endothelial cells and inflammatory cells serve as internal controls and show positive nuclear staining (original magnification, ×400).

at most centers. Although a vast majority (approximately 98%) of AT/RTs exhibit inactivation of SMARCB1 (INI1, hSNF5, and BAF47), a small subgroup of tumors bears an alternative signature, inactivation of SMARCA4 (BRG1), and testing for this abnormality is recommended for those rare cases of AT/RT that do not show SMARCB1/INI1 inactivation.[32]

EMBRYONAL TUMORS WITH MULTILAYERED ROSETTES

The group of embryonal tumors other than medulloblastoma and AT/RT is classified under the generic category, CNS PNETs, in the most recent edition of the WHO classification scheme.[1] This group comprises a diverse category of tumors, likely representing more than 1 specific entity, and includes

- Neuroblastoma
- Ganglioneuroblastoma
- Medulloepithelioma
- Ependymoblastoma
- Embryonal tumors that are not otherwise specified (CNS PNETs, NOS)
- Tumors reported by Eberhart and colleagues[33] as embryonal tumor with abundant neuropil and true rosettes (ETANTR) were also considered in this category as a putative unique variant or entity.

Although there have been many attempts to characterize each of these entities, there are many uncertainties, overlaps, and lack of consensus criteria for the diagnosis of some of these tumors.

Recently, molecular and pathologic analyses of some tumors in this category revealed a common thread that nearly warrants them to be considered in the same entity. A genomic amplification involving the microRNA cluster at the 19q13.42 locus was identified in a case of ETANTR in 2009.[34] Subsequently, the same genetic alteration was discovered in a group of tumors with ependymoblastic rosettes.[35] Finally, most recent reports demonstrated the same genetic signature in ependymoblastomas, medulloepitheliomas, and ETANTR, linking these 3 tumors genetically and clinically into a single clinicopathologic entity.[36,37] The argument in favor of this suggestion is the same genetic alteration in the same locus along with occurrence in the very young and dismal prognosis, resulting in the putative entity, embryonal tumors with multilayered rosettes (ETMRs).[37] These tumors occurred equally among male and female patients, and had a median age of 3 years at presentation. Most examples were supratentorial and typically recurred rapidly during the follow-up period with high rate of mortality and an overall survival of less than 13 months. Currently, demographic features and other characteristics of these tumors are not well established due to very small numbers reported in clinical series. The unifying characteristics of these tumors, however, suggest an aggressive growth and poor prognosis in this young age group with large, solid, and cystic cerebral tumors (Fig. 4A, B).

HISTOPATHOLOGIC FEATURES OF EMBRYONAL TUMORS WITH MULTILAYERED ROSETTES

Based on current understanding, ETMRs are tumors showing a biphasic pattern featuring markedly cellular areas composed of small, blue, round cells typical of primitive blast cells with numerous mitoses and apoptosis admixed with paucicellular, neuropil-rich areas that also contain the same blast cells to a much lesser extent (see Fig. 4C, D). The latter may contain large, more differentiated neuronal cells, also suggested as part of the neoplasm. The tumor is characterized by numerous, multilayered rosettes composed of the same small cells that show marked anaplastic nuclear features, mitosis, and apoptosis. The amount of neuropil varied from tumor to tumor as well as in different parts of the tumor. The tumors with almost no neuropil but with the same hypercellularity and multilayered rosettes were considered in the ependymoblastoma category, because the rosettes were interpreted as primitive ependymal or ependymoblastic (see Fig. 4E). The medulloepithelioma pattern, on the other hand, was predominantly composed of tubular, papillary, trabecular, or even glandular-appearing arrangement of primitive cells that often contain an outer layer reminiscent of the primitive neural tube (see Fig. 4F). Tumors previously classified as medulloepithelioma also contained highly cellular areas with the typical multilayered rosettes. Recent studies also suggested that recurrent tumors that had the typical histologic characteristics of ETANTR in the original tissue transformed into more cellular, ependymoblastoma-like tumors with almost complete loss of neuropil-like areas and also demonstrated papillary of tubular areas reminiscent of medulloepithelioma.[37]

MOLECULAR FEATURES OF EMBRYONAL TUMORS WITH MULTILAYERED ROSETTES

As discussed previously, the most salient molecular feature of these tumors was reported to be amplification of the 19q13.42 region confirmed by different groups.[35,36,38] An earlier study has suggested that amplification of C19MC microRNA polycistron at 19q13.41 was seen in approximately one-quarter of tumors classified as CNS PNETs.[38] These investigators have classified the tumors as CNS PNETs but provided little detail on the histopathologic features, raising the possibility that the tumors identified as having this amplification could also be ETMRs. Subsequently, other investigators found C19MC cluster amplification the most common in tumors classified as ETMRs.[37,39,40] Many of these tumors, approximately three-quarters, also demonstrated gain of chromosome 2, but this was not considered of consequence. Other low-level copy number variations included gain of 7q, 11q, and 1q and loss of 6q.[37]

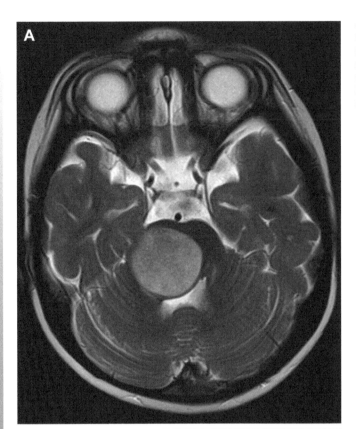

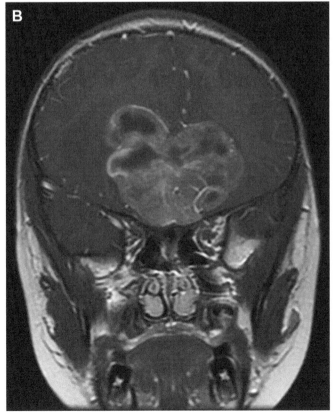

Fig. 4. (*A*) Axial T2-weighted image of an ETMR in the posterior fossa demonstrating a well-defined hyperintense mass in an infant. (*B*) Coronal contrast-enhanced T1-weighted image of an ETMR with histologic features of ependymoblastoma.

Fig. 4. (continued). (*C*) Histologic features of tumors previously designated ETANTRs with neuropil background and multiple multilayered rosettes (original magnification, ×100). (*D*) High-power magnification of the multilayered rosette with marked nuclear anaplasia, mitoses, and apoptosis (original magnification, ×400).

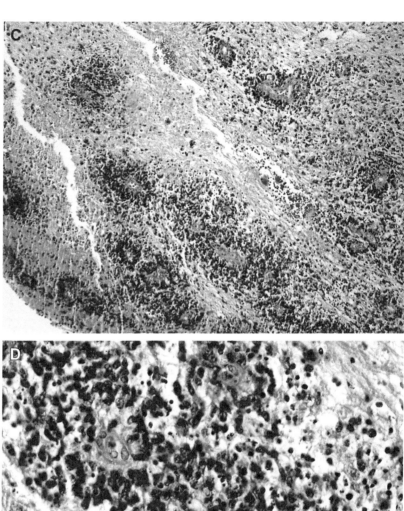

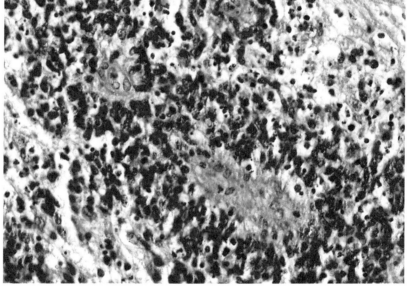

The unique amplicon at 19q13.42 seems to be a 0.89-MB segment that covers the C19MC locus, which harbors a cluster of microRNA-coding genes. This alteration has been suggested as a driver oncogenic event that leads to tumorigenesis in ETMRs.[37] Although this hypothesis seems plausible, it remains to be determined whether it is really the driver oncogenic alteration. Subsequently,

Kleinman and colleagues[40] identified a fusion between TTYH1 and the microRNA cluster in ETMRs. The former is a member of the Tweety family and encodes a chlorine channel that is restricted to neural tissue. It is expressed in almost all embryonal stem cells and embryonal and adult neural tissues. The fusion with TTYH1 was suggested as explaining the brain specificity of tumors harboring the

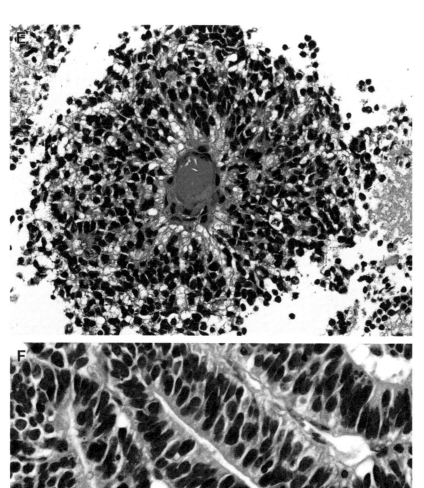

Fig. 4. (continued). (E) High-power magnification of perivascular arrangement in tumors previously reported as ependymoblastoma (original magnification, ×400). (F) High-power magnification of medulloepithelioma features (original magnification, ×400).

C19MC amplification as well as the high levels seen in these tumors. These investigators suggested that the fusion of TTYH1 and C19MC leads to over-expression of this microRNA cluster, leading to abnormal maintenance of chromatin through aberrant expression of brain-specific form of DNMT3B, a de novo methyltransferase gene.[40] This hypothesis implies an oncogenic rearrangement of an embryonal developmental program leading to ETMRs.

A recent immunohistochemical marker, LIN28A, has been identified as a diagnostic marker for ETMRs through high throughput expression analysis.[35] This marker has been found diffusely and intensely positive in the multilayered rosettes and the small, blue, round cells of ETMRs (see Fig. 4D). The staining was less intense in the neuropil-like component. This strong staining could not be detected in many other glial or embryonal tumors, such as medulloblastoma or AT/RT, making it a reliable diagnostic marker for ETMRs. The combination of diffuse, widespread positive LIN28A staining and 19q13.42 amplification seems diagnostic for this putative entity.[37] It is highly likely that this concept will be adopted in the next version of the WHO classification scheme.

REFERENCES

1. Louis DN, Ohgaki H, Wiestler OD, et al. WHO classification of tumors of the central nervous system. 4th edition. Lyon (France): International Agency for Research on Cancer (IARC); 2007.

2. Bailey P, Cushing H. A classification of the tumors of the glioma group on a histogenetic basis with a correlated study of prognosis. Philadelphia; London: J.B. Lippincott Company; 1926.

3. Bailey P. Intracranial tumors. Springfield (IL); Baltimore (MD): C.C. Thomas; 1933.

4. Cushing H. Intracranial tumours. Springfield (IL); Baltimore (MD): C. C. Thomas; 1932.

5. Zülch KJ. Histological typing of tumours of the central nervous system, vol. 21. Geneva (Switzerland): World Health Organization; 1979.

6. Zülch KJ. Brain tumors, their biology and pathology. American edition. New York: Springer Pub Co; 1957.

7. Kleihues P, Burger PC, Scheithauer BW. The new WHO classification of brain tumours. Brain Pathol 1993;3(3):255–68.

8. Kleihues P, Cavenee WK. Pathology and genetics of tumours of the nervous system. World health organization classification of tumours. Lyon (France): IARC Press; 2000.

9. Brown HG, Kepner JL, Perlman EJ, et al. "Large cell/anaplastic" medulloblastomas: a Pediatric Oncology Group Study. J Neuropathol Exp Neurol 2000; 59(10):857–65.

10. Giangaspero F, Rigobello L, Badiali M, et al. Large-cell medulloblastomas. A distinct variant with highly aggressive behavior. Am J Surg Pathol 1992;16(7): 687–93.

11. Lamont JM, McManamy CS, Pearson AD, et al. Combined histopathological and molecular cytogenetic stratification of medulloblastoma patients. Clin Cancer Res 2004;10(16):5482–93.

12. Edelstein K, Spiegler BJ, Fung S, et al. Early aging in adult survivors of childhood medulloblastoma: long-term neurocognitive, functional, and physical outcomes. Neuro Oncol 2011;13(5):536–45.

13. Palmer SL, Hassall T, Evankovich K, et al. Neurocognitive outcome 12 months following cerebellar mutism syndrome in pediatric patients with medulloblastoma. Neuro Oncol 2010;12(12):1311–7.

14. Lafay-Cousin L, Bouffet E, Hawkins C, et al. Impact of radiation avoidance on survival and neurocognitive outcome in infant medulloblastoma. Curr Oncol 2009;16(6):21–8.

15. Batra SK, McLendon RE, Koo JS, et al. Prognostic implications of chromosome 17p deletions in human medulloblastomas. J Neurooncol 1995;24(1): 39–45.

16. Scheurlen WG, Schwabe GC, Joos S, et al. Molecular analysis of childhood primitive neuroectodermal tumors defines markers associated with poor outcome. J Clin Oncol 1998;16(7):2478–85.

17. Ellison DW, Onilude OE, Lindsey JC, et al. Beta-Catenin status predicts a favorable outcome in childhood medulloblastoma: the United Kingdom Children's Cancer Study Group Brain Tumour Committee. J Clin Oncol 2005;23(31):7951–7.

18. Jones DT, Jager N, Kool M, et al. Dissecting the genomic complexity underlying medulloblastoma. Nature 2012;488(7409):100–5.

19. Gottardo NG, Hansford JR, McGlade JP, et al. Medulloblastoma down under 2013: a report from the third annual meeting of the International Medulloblastoma Working Group. Acta Neuropathol 2014; 127(2):189–201.

20. Yachnis AT, Perry A. Embryonal (primitive) neoplasms of the central nervous system. In: Perry A, Brat DJ, editors. Practical surgical neuropathology: a diagnostic approach. Philadelphia: PA: Churchill Livingstone; 2010. p. 165–84.

21. Ellison DW, Dalton J, Kocak M, et al. Medulloblastoma: clinicopathological correlates of SHH, WNT, and non-SHH/WNT molecular subgroups. Acta Neuropathol 2011;121(3):381–96.

22. Gibson P, Tong Y, Robinson G, et al. Subtypes of medulloblastoma have distinct developmental origins. Nature 2010;468(7327):1095–9.

23. Northcott PA, Korshunov A, Witt H, et al. Medulloblastoma comprises four distinct molecular variants. J Clin Oncol 2011;29(11):1408–14.

24. de Haas T, Hasselt N, Troost D, et al. Molecular risk stratification of medulloblastoma patients based on immunohistochemical analysis of MYC, LDHB, and CCNB1 expression. Clin Cancer Res 2008;14(13): 4154–60.

25. Shih DJ, Northcott PA, Remke M, et al. Cytogenetic Prognostication Within Medulloblastoma Subgroups. J Clin Oncol 2014;32(9):886–96.

26. Schwalbe EC, Williamson D, Lindsey JC, et al. DNA methylation profiling of medulloblastoma allows robust subclassification and improved outcome prediction using formalin-fixed biopsies. Acta Neuropathol 2013;125(3):359–71.

27. Hovestadt V, Remke M, Kool M, et al. Robust molecular subgrouping and copy-number profiling of medulloblastoma from small amounts of archival tumour material using high-density DNA methylation arrays. Acta Neuropathol 2013;125(6):913–6.

28. Rorke LB, Packer R, Biegel J. Central nervous system atypical teratoid/rhabdoid tumors of infancy and childhood. J Neurooncol 1995;24(1):21–8.

29. Biegel JA, Tan L, Zhang F, et al. Alterations of the hSNF5/INI1 gene in central nervous system atypical teratoid/rhabdoid tumors and renal and extrarenal rhabdoid tumors. Clin Cancer Res 2002;8(11): 3461–7.

30. Shonka NA, Armstrong TS, Prabhu SS, et al. Atypical teratoid/rhabdoid tumors in adults: a case report and treatment-focused review. J Clin Med Res 2011; 3(2):85–92.

31. Burger PC, Yu IT, Tihan T, et al. Atypical teratoid/ rhabdoid tumor of the central nervous system: a highly malignant tumor of infancy and childhood frequently mistaken for medulloblastoma: a Pediatric Oncology Group study. Am J Surg Pathol 1998; 22(9):1083–92.

32. Hasselblatt M, Gesk S, Oyen F, et al. Nonsense mutation and inactivation of SMARCA4 (BRG1) in an atypical teratoid/rhabdoid tumor showing retained SMARCB1 (INI1) expression. Am J Surg Pathol 2011;35(6):933–5.

33. Eberhart CG, Brat DJ, Cohen KJ, et al. Pediatric neuroblastic brain tumors containing abundant neuropil and true rosettes. Pediatr Dev Pathol 2000;3(4): 346–52.

34. Pfister SM, Korshunov A, Kool M, et al. Molecular diagnostics of CNS embryonal tumors. Acta Neuropathol 2010;120(5):553–66.

35. Korshunov A, Remke M, Gessi M, et al. Focal genomic amplification at 19q13.42 comprises a powerful diagnostic marker for embryonal tumors with ependymoblastic rosettes. Acta Neuropathol 2010;120(2):253–60.

36. Nobusawa S, Yokoo H, Hirato J, et al. Analysis of chromosome 19q13.42 amplification in embryonal brain tumors with ependymoblastic multilayered rosettes. Brain Pathol 2012;22(5):689–97.

37. Korshunov A, Sturm D, Ryzhova M, et al. Embryonal tumor with abundant neuropil and true rosettes (ETANTR), ependymoblastoma, and medulloepithelioma share molecular similarity and comprise a single clinicopathological entity. Acta Neuropathol 2014;128(2):279–89.

38. Li M, Lee KF, Lu Y, et al. Frequent amplification of a chr19q13.41 microRNA polycistron in aggressive primitive neuroectodermal brain tumors. Cancer Cell 2009;16(6):533–46.

39. Nobusawa S, Hirato J. Embryonal tumors with ependymoblastic rosettes-reply. Hum Pathol 2014;45(3): 658.

40. Kleinman CL, Gerges N, Papillon-Cavanagh S, et al. Fusion of TTYH1 with the C19MC microRNA cluster drives expression of a brain-specific DNMT3B isoform in the embryonal brain tumor ETMR. Nat Genet 2014;46(1):39–44.

Recent Developments in Paraneoplastic Disorders of the Nervous System

S. Humayun Gultekin, MD

KEYWORDS

• Neurologic • Autoimmunity • Paraneoplastic disorders • Antibody

ABSTRACT

P araneoplastic disorders of the nervous system (PNDs) are rare and unique disorders, where a specific pattern of neural damage occurs as a side effect of the interaction between the neoplasm and the host immune response. Clinical recognition of PNDs may be challenging but can lead to early detection of an occult neoplasm. Their study may lead to a better understanding of nervous system autoimmunity and even to devising novel immunotherapies against certain tumor types. Familiarity with the clinical syndromes, neuroradiological findings, autoantibodies, and tissue responses associated with PND may help arrive at a correct diagnosis in most cases.

OVERVIEW

Paraneoplastic disorders of the nervous system (PNDs) are rare and unique disorders, where a specific pattern of neural damage occurs as a side effect of the interaction between the neoplasm and the host immune response.[1] Paraneoplastic syndromes where direct and primary damage occurs in the non-neural tissues (hypercalcemia, Trousseau syndrome, and so forth) are excluded here, and discussion is confined it to those that directly affect the nervous system in isolation with a probable autoimmune mechanism. Clinical recognition of PNDs may be challenging but can lead to early detection of an occult neoplasm.[2] PNDs can also be seen as the human body's own "cancer immunotherapy attempt" with variable success and side effects. Their study may lead to a better understanding of nervous system autoimmunity and even to devising novel immunotherapies against certain tumor types.

Pathologists may occasionally encounter a brain biopsy or an autopsy where the differential diagnosis includes PND. Familiarity with the clinical syndromes, neuroradiologic findings, autoantibodies, and tissue responses associated with PND may help arrive at a correct diagnosis in most cases.

CLINICAL SYNDROMES

Any part of the nervous system, from the cerebral neocortex down to the neuromuscular junction and muscle, and the autonomic nervous system can be involved in PNDs. Therefore, clinical involvement pattern may be atypical and variegated, and the differential diagnosis may be broad in individual patients, including viral encephalitis and prion disease. If a patient has a known cancer, PNDs may become more of a possibility but should still be a diagnosis of exclusion.[2]

A typical scenario for a PND patient is a patient with increased risk for cancer who comes to clinical attention with subacute progressive neurologic dysfunction affecting different areas of the nervous system. In approximately one-third of the patients, a previously diagnosed cancer exists, but a majority have no previous history of tumor.[1,2]

Through decades of clinical and laboratory correlation, associations between clinical syndromes, tumor types, and autoantibodies have been identified (Table 1).[3–5] Novel associations are being observed and published every year, however, and atypical syndromes and antibodies have been documented.[6] A useful proposed clinical distinction is between classical and nonclassical paraneoplastic syndromes,[7] where encephalomyelitis, limbic encephalitis, subacute cerebellar degeneration, opsoclonus-myoclonus syndrome, subacute sensory neuronopathy, intestinal

Department of Pathology, Oregon Health & Science University, 3181 SW Sam Jackson Park Road, Portland, OR 97239, USA
E-mail address: gultekin@ohsu.edu

Surgical Pathology 8 (2015) 89–99
http://dx.doi.org/10.1016/j.path.2014.10.005
1875-9181/15/$ – see front matter © 2015 Elsevier Inc. All rights reserved.

surgpath.theclinics.com

Table 1
Paraneoplastic disorders of the nervous system: antibodies, syndromes, neoplasms, and target antigens

Antibody	Syndrome	Neoplasms	Target Antigens
Anti-Hu (ANNA-1)	PEM/DRN	SCLC, neuroblastoma	HuD, HuC, Hel-N1
Anti-Yo (PCA-1)	Cerebellar degeneration	Breast, müllerian	CDR2, CDR2L
Anti-PCA2	PCD, LEMS, PN, encephalitis	SCLC	280 kDa
Anti-Ri (ANNA-2)	BSE, PCD, OM	Breast	Nova
Anti-Ma1	LE, BSE	Lung, other	40-kDa subnuclear
Anti-Ma2 (Ta)	BSE, LE, hypothalamic	Testicular germ cell T.	41.5-kDa subnuclear
Anti-Tr	PCD	Hodgkin lymphoma	DNER
Antiamphiphysin	Stiff person, PEM, PM	Breast, SCLC	Amphiphysin
Antirecoverin	Retinopathy	SCLC, müllerian	Recoverin
Anti-TRPM-1 (bipolar cells)	Retinopathy	Melanoma	Transient receptor potential melastatin 1
Anti-SOX1	LEMS	SCLC	SOX1
Anti-CV2/CRMP5	PEM, PCD, chorea, SN, PM	SCLC, thymoma	CV2/CRMP5
Anti-NMDAR	Encephalitis	Teratoma	NMDAR
Anti-GABA (B)	Limbic encephalitis	SCLC	GABA B1
Anti-mGluR5	LE (Ophelia syndrome)	Hodgkin lymphoma	mGluR5
Anti-mGluR1	Cerebellar ataxia	Hodgkin lymphoma	mGluR1
Anti-LGI1	LE, myoclonus, hyponatremia, seizures	Thymoma	LGI1
Anti-AMPAR	LE, psychosis	Lung, breast, thymus	AMPAR Glu1/2 su
Anti-AChR	Myasthenia gravis	Thymoma	AChR
Anti-AChR-G	Autonomic neuropathy	SCLC, other	Ganglionic AChR
Anti-VGCC	LEMS	SCLC	VGCC
anti–NXP-2, anti–TIF1γ, anti-TIF1α	Dermatomyositis	Colon, lung, breast	NXP-2, TIF1γ, TIF1α
Anti-CASPR2	Morvan syndrome, encephalitis	Thymoma, SCLC	CASPR2
Anti-MAG	Peripheral neuropathy	Waldenström MG	MAG
Anti-GAD65	Stiff person syndrome	Breast, thyroid, other	GAD 65-kDa isoform

Abbreviations: AchR, acetylcholine receptor; AMPAR, AMPA receptor; BSE, brainstem encephalitis; DRN, dorsal root neuronopathy; GAD, glutamic acid decarboxylase; LE, limbic encephalitis; MG, macroglobulinemia; mGluR, metabotropic glutamate receptor; OM, opsoclonus-myoclonus; PCD, paraneoplastic cerebellar degeneration; PEP, paraneoplastic encephalomyelitis; PM, paraneoplastic myelitis; PN, peripheral neuropathy; SN, sensory neuropathy.
    Data from Refs.[3–5]

pseudo-obstruction, Lambert-Eaton myasthenic syndrome (LEMS), and dermatomyositis are considered as the classic paraneoplastic syndromes. These are more likely to be associated with a neoplasm, even when no onconeural antibody is found in patient sera. Metabolic, toxic, infectious, other autoimmune, vascular, and metastatic etiologies should, however, still be eliminated.

AUTOIMMUNE ENCEPHALITIS AND CANCER

Novel associations between clinical encephalitic syndromes, and serologic presence of neuronal surface antibodies with or without underlying cancer have been developed in recent years. The classic paraneoplastic encephalitis syndromes (eg, limbic encephalitis with small cell lung cancer [SCLC]) occur more frequently in older adults, are more likely to herald an underlying neoplasm, are clinically typically uniphasic with variable stabilization, and are limited in their response to therapy. As opposed to the classic PNDs, these recently characterized autoimmune encephalitis (AIE) syndromes are generally more common, occur in younger age groups, respond more frequently to therapy, and may show relapses.[8]

The definition and foundational work for the treatable AIE, anti–N-methyl-D-aspartate receptor encephalitis (Dalmau encephalitis), has been done within the past 10 years by Dalmau and colleagues,[9–11] with in-depth characterization of the clinical syndrome, autoantibody association, pathogenesis, and therapy. Rapid onset of marked behavioral symptoms, seizures, memory impairment, decreased consciousness, and orofacial dyskinesias characterize this entity. Patients are often initially clinically considered as psychiatric patients. In days to weeks, autonomic and respiratory instability ensues. The cerebrospinal fluid (CSF) shows increased lymphocytes and protein elevation. A minority of adult patients show a characteristic electroencephalograhic pattern, called *extreme delta brush*, that may also correlate with disease activity. Cerebral MRI may show nonspecific fluid-attenuated inversion recovery or T2 changes or transient contrast enhancement. Patients also show a relative gradient of glucose metabolism from frontotemporal to the occipital regions when studied by fludeoxyglucose F 18–positron emission tomography (PET). This pattern also disappears with recovery. All patients harbor antibodies against the GluN1 subunit of the N-methyl-D-aspartate receptor (NMDAR) in the serum and/or CSF. The chance of finding an underlying neoplasm is approximately 50%. Many young female patients above the age of 18 with this syndrome harbor ovarian teratomas, which should be found and removed promptly to decrease the risk of relapse and increase the chance of recovery. When these patients are rapidly diagnosed and receive a combination of tumor therapy, first-line immunotherapy, and second-line immunotherapy when necessary, the 2-year outcomes are invariably good.[12] Testing both serum and CSF during initial antibody assays increases the diagnostic yield, because CSF antibodies are procont in all patients, and establishes a baseline to demonstrate decreasing CSF antibody titers in response to therapy.

AIE may constitute a significant percentage of encephalitis cases.[13] Yet, distinguishing viral, autoimmune, and other causes of encephalitis may be challenging in individual patients. Viral encephalitis and AIE cases may have overlapping CSF and MRI findings. Most febrile cases are infectious, with less than 5% of cases eventually diagnosed with an AIE, such as the anti-NMDAR encephalitis.[14] Recognition of typical psychiatric/neurologic symptoms and signs of AIE may be helpful to initiate antibody studies and rapidly institute therapy. Titulaer and colleagues,[12] in a review of 577 patients, observe that more 87% of the anti-NMDAR encephalitis patients develop at least 4 or more of the

following 8 symptom categories within 1 month of onset: psychiatric features, memory disturbance, speech disorder, seizures, dyskinesias, decreased level of consciousness, autonomic instability, and hypoventilation.

In anti-NMDAR encephalitis patients, a clinically confusing overlap may occur. A subset of patients may develop clinical or MRI findings of a demyelinating disorder, concurrent with or independent of the anti-NMDAR encephalitis, with resistance to treatment. Conversely, patients with neuromyelitis optica and other demyelinating disorders with atypical clinical presentation (such as psychiatric, autonomic symptoms and dyskinesias) may be harboring anti–N-methyl-D-aspartate (NMDA) antibodies.[15] An additional association is when patients develop anti-NMDAR encephalitis after a known herpes simplex encephalitis episode. The distinction of herpes simplex encephalitis relapse versus a novel onset of anti-NMDAR encephalitis is critical because immunotherapy must be initiated in the latter.[16]

Other types of neuronal surface antibodies have been identified in patients with AIE-type clinical syndrome. These have various antigenic targets, such as α-amino-3-hydroxy-5-methyl-4-isoxazolepropionic acid (AMPA), γ-aminobutyric acid (GABA), glutamine receptor subtypes, leucine-rich glioma inactivated 1 (LGI1), dipeptidyl-peptidase–like protein 6 (DPPX), and contactin-associated protein 2 (CASPR2).[17] They may show variable involvement of other parts of the nervous system with or without limbic symptoms. These may variably be associated with cancer (lung, breast, or thymus cancer; Hodgkin lymphoma; SCLC; and so forth) and other autoimmune diseases.

A notable development has been the recent identification of LGI1 as the main target antigen in nonparaneoplastic autoimmune limbic encephalitis cases,[18] in which the autoantibody was previously thought to be against voltage-gated potassium channels (VGKCs).[19] The previous misidentification was due to coimunoprecipitation of the VGKC with LGI1 with the commercially available assay used. Feline complex partial seizures with orofacial involvement cases also have been shown associated with these antibodies, and the neuropathologic findings are similar to those of humans, with hippocampal T-cell infiltrates with IgG and C9neo deposits and neuronal loss.[20]

Another recent development has been the identification of delta/notch-like epidermal growth factor–related receptor (DNER) as the target antigen in paraneoplastic cerebellar degeneration associated with Hodgkin lymphoma (anti-Tr). The main epitope was identified within the extracellular domain of DNER, and N-glycosylation of the

DNER turned out to be the critical element in recognition of this epitope by anti-Tr sera.[21] Another recently identified autoantigen is the target of paraneoplastic encephalitis in Hodgkin lymphoma (Ophelia syndrome) as the mGluR5.[22] In an anti-Hu negative group of limbic encephalitis patients, the SCLC patients have been discovered to harbor GABA(B) receptor antibodies, a more treatment-responsive group.[23] Another GABA receptor subtype, GABA(A) has recently been identified as the target protein in a group of patients with encephalitis with refractory seizures and status epilepticus without underlying neoplasm—a potentially treatable disorder.[24]

MECHANISMS OF DISEASE

The main proposed pathogenetic mechanism is based on an interaction between the neoplastic tissue and the immune system. The host develops an autoimmune reaction against often aberrantly expressed neural or neuroendocrine tumoral protein antigens, which attack both the tumor and the host neural tissues that share the antigen.

Response to immunosuppressive therapy and plasmapheresis and passive serum transfer studies successfully reproducing most of the symptoms in mice support an antibody-mediated pathogenesis in LEMS, associated with P/Q-type voltage-gated calcium channel (VGCC) antibodies, as well as in myasthenia gravis associated with thymoma. Similarly, for most encephalitic PNDs with neuronal surface receptor proteins as target antigens, there are experimental data that the presence of antibody may play a pathogenetic role. In limbic encephalitis, the actual target of VGKC antibodies is Lgi1, a protein involved in excitatory synaptic transmission.[18] In anti-NMDAR encephalitis, the antibodies seem to block the extracellular epitopes of the NR1 subunit, hence creating a relative predominance of glutamatergic activity. Antibodies cause decreased levels of synaptic NMDAR and reversibly disrupt NMDAR-dependent synaptic currents in cultured neurons.[25,26] The more recent studies on rodent brains using anti-NMDAR antibodies support an immunoglobulin-induced receptor internalization.[27] Tüzün and colleagues[28] found markedly increased microglia, sparse perivascular B-cell and rare parenchymal T-cell infiltrates, and diffuse IgG deposits in autopsy brains of anti-NMDAR encephalitis, without significant neuronal death and without complement deposition. A subsequent study of autopsy/biopsy tissues and teratomas of a larger patient group found perivascular T and B cells as well as numerous plasma cells but no complement deposits in patient brain tissues as opposed to the neural tissues of patient teratomas.[29] Combined with response to therapy and CSF findings, all these studies point to a humoral-based pathogenesis in NMDAR encephalitis.

The onconeural antigens that are associated with the classic PNDs, such as Hu, Yo, Ri, and CRMP5, are intracellular. These antibodies are apparently unable to access these target antigens that do not have a surface presence. The immune response in the associated PND seems to be predominantly cytotoxic T-cell mediated.[30] Direct pathogenetic role of the associated serum and CSF antibodies has not been shown in any of these syndromes. A recent report, however, states that CDR2L, one of the anti-Yo syndrome antibodies, localizes to the cell membrane as well as to the cytoplasm with confocal microscopy.[31] This shows that theories on pathogenesis will evolve as more about the biology of these antigens and the host immune response is learned. Studying tissues that belong to an early stage of the disease process may also be more valuable to derive more reliable information out of tissue-based immunopathogenetic studies.

A smaller third group of antibodies, whose target antigens are intracellular synaptic proteins, such as GAD65 and amphiphysin, is associated with stiff person syndrome. There is some evidence, however, that these proteins may have an extracellular domain, or the antigens may be exposed on the cell surface during synaptic vesicle recycling. GAD65-sensitized T cells can cause encephalomyelitis when transferred to GAD65-naïve mice.[32] Passive transfer of antiamphiphysin IgG also results in stiffness and myospasms in mice.[33]

Host factors also may play a role in the development of PND. Some cancer patients with serum onconeural antibodies do not become symptomatic. Major histocompatibility complex (MHC) haplotypes and tumor-specific factors may also be important. PND-associated tumors often show marked lymphocytic infiltrates under the microscope. One of the most obscure aspects of the pathophysiology of PND is how the peripheral immune response is translated into a central nervous system (CNS) immune response in the presence of the blood-brain barrier. Tumor cell apoptosis may induce immunogenicity. Thymic factors, such as AIRE mutations in thymic epithelial cells that regulate tolerance to peripheral tissue-restricted antigens may also contribute to the individualization of the immune response and development of autoimmunity in cancer.[34] Tumor-associated regulatory T cells may be undergoing a development stage in the thymus via an AIRE-dependent process.[35]

LABORATORY DIAGNOSIS OF PARANEOPLASTIC DISORDERS OF THE NERVOUS SYSTEM

RADIOLOGY

An initial normal cerebral MRI is common. Significant contrast enhancement is unusual in PNDs (Fig. 1). Different modalities are useful to eliminate other causes. Both cerebral and spinal MRI may be useful to show extent and pattern of involvement. Cerebral or cerebellar atrophy may be detected in long-standing cases.

CEREBROSPINAL FLUID

Lymphocytic pleocytosis, elevated protein, and oligoclonal bands can be found in a majority of patients but rarely the CSF may be completely normal.

SEROLOGY

Detection of high-titer antibodies against intracellular antigens (Hu, Yo, CRMP5, and amphiphysin) is highly specific for PND. Detection of antibodies against neuronal surface antigens can be associated with underlying cancer or may be idiopathic.

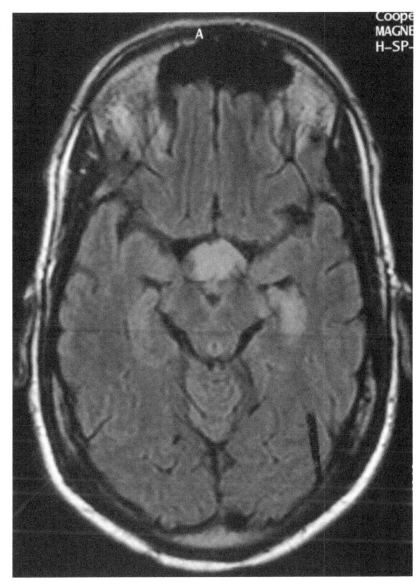

Fig. 1. Cerebral MRI of a patient with limbic encephalitis.

There are rare seronegative cases. The testing should be performed in both serum and CSF, when available.

Antibody detection methods have different yield depending on the antibody type. Tissue-based assays are better for the intracellular antigens. They are based on the demonstration of serum antigens on fresh rat brain histologic sections via immunohistochemical (IHC) methods. Relevant brain regions, such as the hippocampus or the cerebellum, are important to include for proper screening. IHC assays on fresh mammalian brain samples are technically difficult and interpretation requires a trained observer. The regions of the brain tissue that are reactive with patient sera and the subcellular compartment of reactivity are important. For example, anti-Hu reactivity consists of intense nuclear staining sparing the nucleolus and moderate cytoplasmic staining confined to the neurons. The anti-Yo antibody labeling is confined to the cerebellar cortex, mostly to Purkinje cells. The anti-NMDA antibody labeling pattern is diffuse neuropil staining, resembling that of a synaptic protein (**Fig. 2**).[36] Presence of multiple autoantibodies may cause additional difficulties in interpretation. Still, IHC

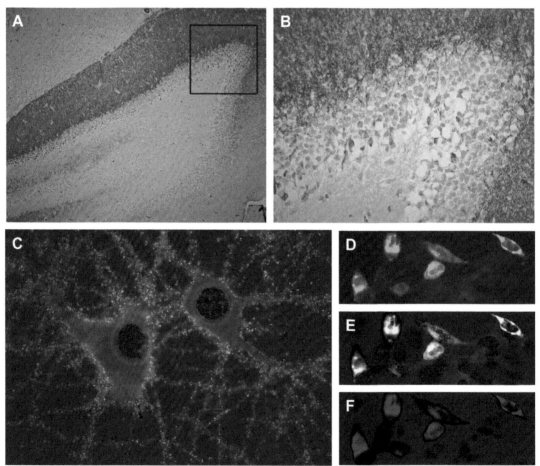

Fig. 2. Demonstration of NMDA receptor antibodies in a patient's CSF. (*A, B*) Sagittal section of rat hippocampus incubated with the patient's CSF (diluted 1:20). The NMDAR antibodies produce intense immunolabeling of the molecular layer, adjacent to the granular cells of the dentate gyrus (faintly counterstained with hematoxylin). (*B*) The area of the dentate gyrus included in the box is shown magnified. (*C*) Cultured rat hippocampal neurons incubated with the patient's CSF demonstrate intense immunolabeling of NMDARs contained in the surface of neurons and neuronal processes (nuclei demonstrated by staining with DAPI). (*D–F*) Confirmation that the CSF antibodies selectively react with NMDARs is shown using human embryonic kidney (HEK293) cells expressing NR1/NR2B heteromers of the NMDAR. The reactivity of the patient's antibodies (*green*) (*D*) colocalize (*yellow*) (*E*) with the reactivity of NR2B-specific antibodies (*red*) (*F*). (*From* Sansing LH, Tüzün E, Ko MW, et al. A patient with encephalitis associated with NMDA receptor antibodies. Nat Clin Pract Neurol 2007;3(5):291–6; with permission from the Nature Publishing Group (UK).)

assays are critical tools for discovery of novel autoantibodies. For previously undescribed antibodies, careful characterization with immunoabsorption, immunoprecipitation, Western blotting, cell-based assays, and mass spectrometry should be used together when possible. Immunoblotting can also be used successfully for detection of most intracellular antigens as a confirmatory test, with the exception of anti-Tr antibody. Commercially prepared blots of the most common onconeural antigens (Hu, Ma, Yo, and so forth) exist. Other than the well-established nitrocellulose membrane-based methods, there are multiplex assays that allow simultaneous testing of multiple antigens, using covalent bonding of antigens to color-coded polystyrene beads.[37] Cell-based assays are the preferred testing method for neuronal surface antigens. They are based on cell lines (for instance, HEK293) transfected with a plasmid containing the encoded target antigen. This material then can be used to screen for the presence of serum/CSF antibodies against this target antigen using an immunofluorescence assay. Commercial plasmids or cell lines are available for the common surface proteins, such as NMDAR and LGI1. ELISA may be helpful to determine antibody titers. Immunoprecipitation may also be used for serum samples and is used to detect mainly VGCC antibodies. A promising recent study suggests that mass spectrometry can be used for detection of antigen-specific immunoglobulin peptides in paraneoplastic patient sera.[38] This approach may eventually be helpful to eliminate some of the more cumbersome assays and to simplify the search for novel antibodies.

The somewhat subjective interpretative nature of IHC and fluorescence-based immunocytochemical assays call for a methodical approach, with strict controls and experience in assays and interpretation. Nonspecific background reactivity, low dilutions of primary antibodies, and low patient antibody titers may be sources for limited sensitivity and specificity. Active intrathecal antibody synthesis in these disorders leads to detectible levels of the antibody in the CSF samples. The CSF antibody titers are more stable and may correlate better with disease activity than serum titers. Using the CSF initially and during follow-up testing usually leads to more reliable results. Correlation of serum and CSF results and using other methods of testing when CSF is negative are important precautions.[39] Optimization of IHC techniques combined with simultaneous use of other detection methods and careful study of tissue distribution/reactivity patterns may increase sensitivity and specificity in autoantibody testing.[40]

SCREENING FOR OCCULT NEOPLASM

If the clinical syndrome is classic and there are high-titer onconeural antibodies, then the probability of a PND is high. Therefore, more aggressive cancer screening can be undertaken. The tests may include mammography, upper and lower gastrointestinal endoscopy, CT and MRI of the abdomen and chest, abdominal/pelvic/transvaginal ultrasonography, and PET. The European Federation of Neurologic Societies Task Force has recently recommended more specific guidelines for individual body sites, cancer types, and tests of choice.[41] If primary screening fails to discover tumor, repeat screening is recommended every 6 months for 4 the next years, except up to 2 years in LEMS.

PATHOLOGY

Central Nervous System Pathology

Brain biopsies may be performed in diagnostically challenging patients, and pathologists may be presented with the differential diagnosis of paraneoplastic disease, vasculitis, viral encephalitis, acute disseminated encephalomyelitis, prion disease, CNS effects of systemic diseases (endocrine or rheumatologic), and so forth. Often, specific diagnosis is elusive in brain biopsies for medical CNS disease, unless a virus or other infectious agent is demonstrated by special stains or there is histologic evidence of frank vasculitis. The histopathologic picture of a PND may be practically indistinguishable from that of a viral encephalitis. Some cases, as in opsoclonus-myoclonus syndrome, may show only perivascular lymphocytic cuffing. Others, especially marked encephalomyelitis cases, show perivascular and parenchymal T-cell infiltrates and widespread neuronal destruction with associated reactive astrogliosis (Fig. 3). Microglial infiltrates are common, and occasional typical microglial nodules may be present. Viral inclusions have not been identified and other viral studies have been negative in CNS tissues of established paraneoplastic syndrome cases. Rasmussen encephalitis may be pathologically similar but typically involves the frontotemporal and peri-insular areas in a single brain hemisphere and spreads to the occipital region with time. There are predominantly neocortical diffuse T-cell infiltrates and microglial nodules, with neuronal destruction and gliosis.

Other recent studies on autopsy/biopsy brain tissues showed some immunopathologic differences among subtypes of autoantibody-associated encephalitis.[42] In the intracellular antigen-onconeural

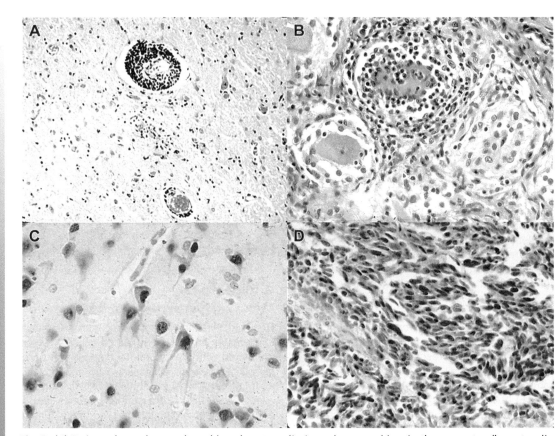

Fig. 3. (*A*) Perivascular and parenchymal lymphocytes, gliosis, and neuronal loss in the neocortex (hematoxylin-eosin, ×100). (*B*) Dorsal root ganglion with lymphocytic infiltrates and loss of ganglion cells (hematoxylin-eosin, ×400). (*C*) Anti-Hu patient serum reacting with normal human brain with IHC, with selective labeling of neuronal nuclei and cytoplasm. DAB light microscopic IHC with patient serum IgG (light hematoxylin counterstaining, ×200). (*D*) SCLC tissue expressing Hu antigens. 3,3'-diaminobenzidine (DAB) light microscopic IHC with patient serum IgG (light hematoxylin counterstaining, ×200).

group (Hu, Ma2), CNS tissues showed a CD8-predominant inflammation with frequently observed granzyme B+ cytotoxic T-cell apposi-tions to neurons expressing MHC-1. In the surface antigen group, the VGKC (LGI1) cases showed complement *C9neo* deposition on neurons associ-ated with acute neuronal cell death, whereas the NMDAR encephalitis cases only low density of in-flammatory cells with no neuronal pathology or complement deposition.

Tumor Pathology

The neoplastic tissues found in PND patients typically grow slower than in nonparaneoplastic patients and may demonstrably regress in size, even vanish. Special attention at autopsy may be necessary to discover an SCLC that may be confined to a single hilar lymph node in an anti-Hu–associated encephalomyelitis case, or careful sectioning of the ovaries may reveal a tiny ovarian carcinoma that would otherwise go undetected in a cerebellar degeneration pa-tient. Under the microscope, most of these neoplastic tissues show marked lymphocytic in-filtrates. The tumor tissues also often react with the patient serum or CSF, and tumor cells can be shown to express the target antigen by IHC or Western blotting. In recently characterized NMDAR encephalitis cases, a predominantly T-cell inflammation was observed in all associ-ated teratoma tissues but not necessarily confined to the neural part of the teratomas. Pa-tient sera IHC labeling pattern in tumor tissues also colocalized with that of commercial anti-bodies against NR1 domain of the NMDA recep-tor complex.[28] Another study of the pathology of ovarian teratomas associated with NMDAR encephalitis described prominent lymphohistio-cytic infiltrates colonizing the neuroglial elements, reactive germinal center formation, and degenerative changes in the neurons in teratoma tissues.[43]

TREATMENT

Rapid institution of standard treatment of the specific cancer has been the most successful therapy for paraneoplastic syndromes. Regression or stabilization of neurologic symptoms, increased life expectancy, and decreased neurologic relapse are among the outcomes with tumor treatment. Other than radiologically or clinically detectable straightforward tumoral lesions, organ removal for suspected microscopic tumor may be performed using strict criteria. A well-characterized clinical situation is when a young man develops limbic encephalitis, anti-Ma antibodies are detected in the serum/CSF,[44,45] and orchiectomy reveals intratubular germ cell neoplasia.[46] In refractory cases, immunomodulatory treatments can be used. These include steroids, steroid-sparing immunosuppressive agents, intravenous immunoglobulin (IVIG), and plasmapheresis. These treatments may also be tried if no underlying neoplasm has been detected. PND associated with neuronal cell membrane antibodies may respond to immunomodulatory treatment more favorably.

As an example of a relatively treatment-responsive group, in confirmed adult anti-NMDAR encephalitis, an initial concurrent methylprednisolone and IVIG therapy should be tried. If not responsive, cyclophosphamide and rituximab can be used. Response to immunotherapy in the pediatric age group is less predictable. Clinical course should be closely monitored for assessing therapy response, and CSF antibody titers may help guide the same.[47] Screening for an underlying neoplasm should be repeated yearly for 2 to 3 years. Increased risk of relapses in a tumor-negative group may warrant azathioprine or mycophenolate mofetil therapy after recovery.[12]

SUMMARY

PNDs are rare but present important diagnostic considerations in various clinical situations. Pathologists should remain aware of the potentially treatable nature of a subset of these disorders. Therefore, during non-neoplastic brain biopsy interpretation, PNDs should be part of their differential diagnostic list in cases with a histopathologic pattern of subacute encephalitis. Conversely, tumors containing unusual inflammatory infiltrates should also alert pathologists to the possibility of a paraneoplastic process in these patients. The recent definition of treatable AIE syndromes exemplified by the NMDAR encephalitis opened new horizons in this field. Recent studies on the association of demyelinating disorders with AIE and the relationship of herpes simplex encephalitis with NMDAR encephalitis bring additional levels of complexity to the accurate diagnosis of individual patients.

REFERENCES

1. Darnell RB, Posner JB. Paraneoplastic syndromes affecting the nervous system. Semin Oncol 2006; 33(3):270–98.
2. Didelot A, Honnorat J. Paraneoplastic disorders of the central and peripheral nervous systems. Handb Clin Neurol 2014;121:1159–79.
3. Rosenfeld MR, Dalmau J. Diagnosis and management of paraneoplastic neurologic disorders. Curr Treat Options Oncol 2013;14(4):528–38.
4. Leypoldt F, Wandinger KP. Paraneoplastic neurological syndromes. Clin Exp Immunol 2014;175(3):336–48.
5. Graus F, Dalmau J. Paraneoplastic neuropathies. Curr Opin Neurol 2013;26(5):489–95.
6. Honnorat J. Onconeural antibodies are essential to diagnose paraneoplastic neurological syndromes. Acta Neurol Scand Suppl 2006;183:64–8.
7. Graus F, Delattre JY, Antoine JC, et al. Recommended diagnostic criteria for paraneoplastic neurological syndromes. J Neurol Neurosurg Psychiatr 2004;75(8):1135–40.
8. Graus F, Dalmau J. Paraneoplastic neurological syndromes. Curr Opin Neurol 2012;25(6):795–801.
9. Dalmau J, Tüzün E, Wu HY, et al. Paraneoplastic anti-N-methyl-D-aspartate receptor encephalitis associated with ovarian teratoma. Ann Neurol 2007;61(1):25–36.
10. Lancaster E, Dalmau J. Neuronal autoantigens–pathogenesis, associated disorders and antibody testing. Nat Rev Neurol 2012;8(7):380–90.
11. Lancaster E, Martinez-Hernandez E, Dalmau J. Encephalitis and antibodies to synaptic and neuronal cell surface proteins. Neurology 2011;77(2):179–89.
12. Titulaer MJ, McCracken L, Gabilondo I, et al. Treatment and prognostic factors for long-term outcome in patients with anti-NMDA receptor encephalitis: an observational cohort study. Lancet Neurol 2013; 12(2):157–65.
13. Armangue T, Leypoldt F, Dalmau J. Autoimmune encephalitis as differential diagnosis of infectious encephalitis. Curr Opin Neurol 2014;27(3):361–8.
14. Thomas L, Mailles A, Desestret V, et al, Steering Committee and Investigators Group. Autoimmune N-methyl-D-aspartate receptor encephalitis is a differential diagnosis of infectious encephalitis. J Infect 2014;68(5):419–25.
15. Titulaer MJ, Höftberger R, Iizuka T, et al. Overlapping demyelinating syndromes and

anti–N-methyl-D-aspartate receptor encephalitis. Ann Neurol 2014;75(3):411–28.

16. Armangue T, Leypoldt F, Málaga I, et al. Herpes simplex virus encephalitis is a trigger of brain autoimmunity. Ann Neurol 2014;75(2):317–23.

17. Dalmau J, Rosenfeld MR. Autoimmune encephalitis update. Neuro Oncol 2014;16(6):771–8.

18. Lai M, Huijbers MG, Lancaster E, et al. Investigation of LGI1 as the antigen in limbic encephalitis previously attributed to potassium channels: a case series. Lancet Neurol 2010;9(8):776–85.

19. Vincent A, Buckley C, Schott JM, et al. Potassium channel antibody-associated encephalopathy: a potentially immunotherapy-responsive form of limbic encephalitis. Brain 2004;127(Pt 3):701–12.

20. Klang A, Schmidt P, Kneissl S, et al. IgG and complement deposition and neuronal loss in cats and humans with epilepsy and voltage-gated potassium channel complex antibodies. J Neuropathol Exp Neurol 2014;73(5):403–13.

21. de Graaff E, Maat P, Hulsenboom E, et al. Identification of delta/notch-like epidermal growth factor-related receptor as the Tr antigen in paraneoplastic cerebellar degeneration. Ann Neurol 2012;71(6):815–24.

22. Lancaster E, Martinez-Hernandez E, Titulaer MJ, et al. Antibodies to metabotropic glutamate receptor 5 in the Ophelia syndrome. Neurology 2011;77(18):1698–701.

23. Lancaster E, Lai M, Peng X, et al. Antibodies to the GABA(B) receptor in limbic encephalitis with seizures: case series and characterisation of the antigen. Lancet Neurol 2010;9(1):67–76.

24. Petit-Pedrol M, Armangue T, Peng X, et al. Encephalitis with refractory seizures, status epilepticus, and antibodies to the GABAA receptor: a case series, characterisation of the antigen, and analysis of the effects of antibodies. Lancet Neurol 2014;13(3):276–86.

25. Dalmau J, Gleichman AJ, Hughes EG, et al. Anti-NMDA-receptor encephalitis: case series and analysis of the effects of antibodies. Lancet Neurol 2008;7(12):1091–8.

26. Hughes EG, Peng X, Gleichman AJ, et al. Cellular and synaptic mechanisms of anti-NMDA receptor encephalitis. J Neurosci 2010;30(17):5866–75.

27. Moscato EH, Peng X, Jain A, et al. Acute mechanisms underlying antibody effects in anti-NMDA receptor encephalitis. Ann Neurol 2014. http://dx.doi.org/10.1002/ana.24195.

28. Tüzün E, Zhou L, Baehring JM, et al. Evidence for antibody-mediated pathogenesis in anti-NMDAR encephalitis associated with ovarian teratoma. Acta Neuropathol 2009;118(6):737–43.

29. Martinez-Hernandez E, Horvath J, Shiloh-Malawsky Y, et al. Analysis of complement and plasma cells in the brain of patients with anti-NMDAR encephalitis. Neurology 2011;77(6):589–93.

30. Pignolet BS, Gebauer CM, Liblau RS. Immunopathogenesis of paraneoplastic neurological syndromes associated with anti-Hu antibodies: a beneficial antitumor immune response going awry. Oncoimmunology 2013;2(12):e27384.

31. Eichler TW, Totland C, Haugen M, et al. CDR2L antibodies: a new player in paraneoplastic cerebellar degeneration. PLoS One 2013;8(6):e66002.

32. Burton AR, Baquet Z, Eisenbarth GS, et al. Central nervous system destruction mediated by glutamic acid decarboxylase-specific CD4+ T cells. J Immunol 2010;184(9):4863–70.

33. Sommer C, Weishaupt A, Brinkhoff J, et al. Paraneoplastic stiff-person syndrome: passive transfer to rats by means of IgG antibodies to amphiphysin. Lancet 2005;365(9468):1406–11.

34. Meager A, Peterson P, Willcox N. Hypothetical review: thymic aberrations and type-I interferons; attempts to deduce autoimmunizing mechanisms from unexpected clues in monogenic and paraneoplastic syndromes. Clin Exp Immunol 2008;154(1):141–51.

35. Malchow S, Leventhal DS, Nishi S, et al. Aire-dependent thymic development of tumor-associated regulatory T cells. Science 2013;339(6124):1219–24.

36. Sansing LH, Tüzün E, Ko MW, et al. A patient with encephalitis associated with NMDA receptor antibodies. Nat Clin Pract Neurol 2007;3(5):291–6.

37. Maat P, Brouwer E, Hulsenboom E, et al. Multiplex serology of paraneoplastic antineuronal antibodies. J Immunol Methods 2013;391(1–2):125–32.

38. Maat P, VanDuijn M, Brouwer E, et al. Mass spectrometric detection of antigen-specific immunoglobulin peptides in paraneoplastic patient sera. J Autoimmun 2012;38(4):354–60.

39. Rosenfeld MR, Titulaer MJ, Dalmau J. Paraneoplastic syndromes and autoimmune encephalitis: five new things. Neurol Clin Pract 2012;2(3):215–23.

40. Höftberger R, Dalmau J, Graus F. Clinical neuropathology practice guide 5-2012: updated guideline for the diagnosis of antineuronal antibodies. Clin Neuropathol 2012;31(5):337–41.

41. Titulaer MJ, Soffietti R, Dalmau J, et al, European Federation of Neurological Societies. Screening for tumours in paraneoplastic syndromes: report of an EFNS task force. Eur J Neurol 2011;18(1):19-e3.

42. Bien CG, Vincent A, Barnett MH, et al. Immunopathology of autoantibody-associated encephalitides: clues for pathogenesis. Brain 2012;135(Pt 5):1622–38.

43. Dabner M, McCluggage WG, Bundell C, et al. Ovarian teratoma associated with anti-N-methyl D-aspartate receptor encephalitis: a report of 5 cases documenting prominent intratumoral lymphoid infiltrates. Int J Gynecol Pathol 2012;31(5):429–37.

44. Gultekin SH, Rosenfeld MR, Voltz R, et al. Paraneoplastic limbic encephalitis: neurological symptoms, immunological findings and tumour association in 50 patients. Brain 2000;123(Pt 7):1481–94.

45. Voltz R, Gultekin SH, Rosenfeld MR, et al. A serologic marker of paraneoplastic limbic and brain-stem encephalitis in patients with testicular cancer. N Engl J Med 1999;340(23):1788–95.

46. Mathew RM, Vandenberghe R, Garcia-Merino A, et al. Orchiectomy for suspected microscopic tumor in patients with anti-Ma2-associated encephalitis. Neurology 2007;68(12):900–5.

47. Gresa-Arribas N, Titulaer MJ, Torrents A, et al. Antibody titres at diagnosis and during follow-up of anti-NMDA receptor encephalitis: a retrospective study. Lancet Neurol 2014;13(2):167–77.

Printed and bound by CPI Group (UK) Ltd, Croydon, CR0 4YY

03/10/2024

01040381-0006